The
Healthy Baby
Meal Planner

200 QUICK, EASY, AND HEALTHY RECIPES
FOR YOUR BABY AND TODDLER

Annabel Karmel

Atria Books
NEW YORK LONDON TORONTO SYDNEY NEW DELHI

This book is dedicated to my children, Nicholas, Lara, and Scarlett, and to the memory of my first daughter, Natasha.

ATRIA BOOKS

A Division of Simon & Schuster, Inc.
1230 Avenue of the Americas
New York, NY 10020

First Atria Books hardcover edition April 2012

ATRIA BOOKS and colophon are trademarks of Simon & Schuster, Inc.

For information about special discounts for bulk purchases, please contact Simon
& Schuster Special Sales at 1-866-506-1949 or business@simonandschuster.com.

The Simon & Schuster Speakers Bureau can bring authors to your live event. For
more information or to book an event, contact the Simon & Schuster Speakers
Bureau at 1-866-248-3049 or visit our website at www.simonspeakers.com.

Design: Smith & Gilmour, London
Illustrations: Nadine Wickenden
Photography: Dave King

Manufactured in China

10 9 8 7 6 5 4 3 2 1

ISBN 978-1-4516-6559-8

Contents

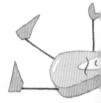

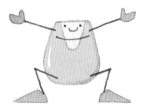

Introduction

Weaning your baby is an exciting milestone for any parent. Unfortunately, as soon as you consult family, friends, websites, and magazines excitement turns to anxiety. You already feel guilty that you started weaning your baby at five months and after two weeks of bland, tasteless baby rice you are wondering whether you should venture into the unknown and purée some carrots. But do they contain nitrates? Should they be organic and do you boil or steam them? Should you give carrots for three days, looking for signs of allergy, before moving on to another food? If you freeze portions in ice-cube trays, should you sterilize the trays first, and is it safe to defrost the cubes in a microwave? And that's just vegetables … When is it safe to give fish, chicken, or meat? Feeding a baby soon becomes a world of wonderment and confusion.

How many old wives' tales have you been told? Do you find yourself withholding foods like eggs, meat, and fish but not really knowing why? I'm sorry to say that a lot of the advice you are given is not based on any scientific research. My aim is to guide you through feeding your baby, taking each stage month by month, separating truth from fiction, answering all your questions – thereby giving you the confidence to prepare fresh food that will give your baby the very best start in life.

In early childhood, eating habits and tastes (good or bad) are formed for life. Babies grow more rapidly in their first year than at any other time and you have this window of opportunity between six and twelve months where you can develop your baby's taste buds. This is the time to introduce many different flavors and textures. Move on to meat, chicken, and fish after a few weeks – these are vitally important foods in the first year – and start mashing and chopping food early on or your child can get lazy about chewing. If you bring up your child on fresh foods from the start, the transition to family meals will be much easier. Miss this crucial time and your child may join the ranks of picky eaters.

I first wrote this book back in 1991 after the untimely death of my first child Natasha, who died due to a rare viral disease. I wanted some good to come from Natasha's short life so I spent many years researching the whole subject of child nutrition, working with top experts in the field. Since its first publication, this has been the leading book on feeding babies and children and has been translated into over 20 languages. This new edition takes in all the latest research in child nutrition, includes new improved versions of the original recipes, 25 brand-new recipes, and photographs that bring the recipes to life.

90 percent of junk food is bought by parents for their kids, and childhood obesity is a growing problem; we need to bring back home cooking. I've probably spent more time in the kitchen cooking up healthy children's meals than almost anyone, and all the recipes are tested on a panel of babies and toddlers. With a little bit of help from the book, you too can be making really nutritious food that's easy to prepare and plate-lickingly good. I can also promise that you and your kids will love the results without spending hours in the kitchen.

I hope you enjoy the advice and recipes in this book as much as I have enjoyed creating them . . .

Annabel Karmel

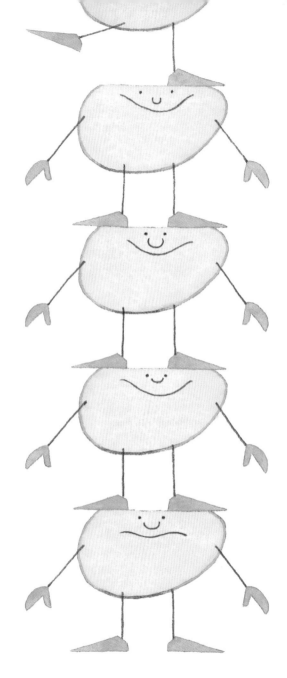

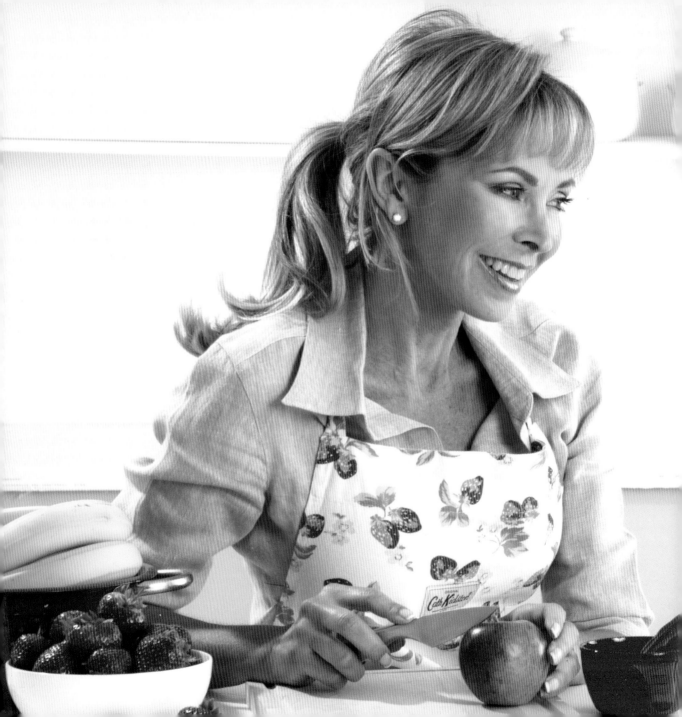

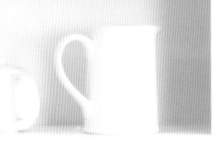

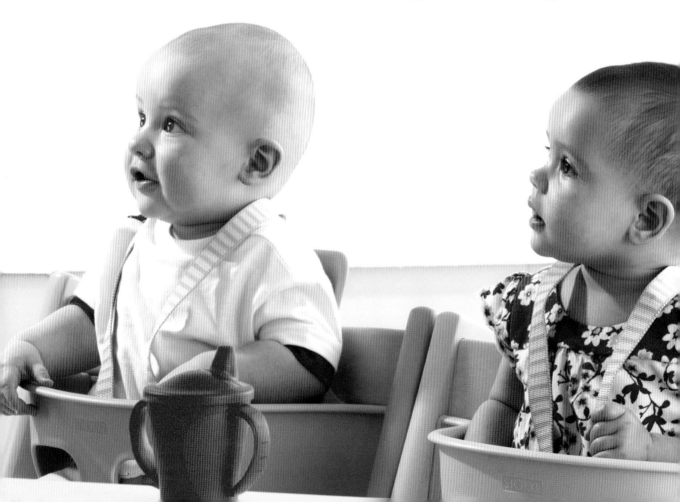

CHAPTER ONE

The best first foods for your baby

The current US Department of Health and Human Services recommendations state that babies should not begin weaning until they are six months old and should be exclusively breastfed until this time. Most babies shouldn't need solid foods before the age of six months, but if you feel that your baby does need them earlier, speak to your pediatrician. Signs that your baby may be ready are listed on page 22. However, the very minimum age for weaning should be 17 weeks, as a baby's digestive system won't fully mature for the first few months and foreign proteins very early on may increase the likelihood of food allergies.

Milk is still the major food

It is very important to remember, when starting to give your baby solid food, that milk is still the best and most natural food for growing babies. I would encourage mothers to give breastfeeding a try. Apart from the emotional benefits, breast milk contains antibodies that will help protect infants from infection. In the first few months babies are particularly vulnerable, and the colostrum a mother produces in the first few days of breastfeeding is a very important source of antibodies, which help to build up a baby's immune system. (If only for this reason, it is obvious that there are some enormous benefits in breastfeeding your child, even for as little as one week.) It is also medically proven that breastfed babies are less likely to develop certain diseases in later life.

Milk should contain all the nutrients your baby needs to grow. There are 65 calories in 4 oz (½ cup) milk, and infant formula milk is fortified with vitamins and iron. Cow's milk isn't such a "complete" food for human babies so is best not started until your baby is one year old. Solids are introduced to add bulk to a baby's diet and to introduce new tastes, textures, and aromas; they also help the baby to practice using the muscles in his mouth. But giving a baby too much solid food too early may lead to constipation and provide fewer nutrients than he needs. It would be very difficult for a baby to get the equivalent amount of nutrients from the small amount of solids he will consume as he gets from his milk.

Don't use softened water or repeatedly boiled water when making up your baby's bottle, because of the danger of concentrating mineral salts. Babies' bottles should not be warmed in a microwave, as the milk may be too hot even though the bottle feels cool to the touch. Warm bottles by standing them in hot water.

Between four and six months, babies should have 21–28 oz (2½–3½ cups) breast milk or infant formula each day (21 oz [2½ cups] is enough once additional solids are introduced, but you'll need to feed more if this is the sole source of your baby's nutrition). It's important to make sure that, up to the age of eight months, your baby drinks milk at least four times a day (especially as it is highly likely that a bottle may not be finished at each feed). If the number of feeds is reduced too quickly, your baby will not be able to drink as much as is needed. Some mothers make the mistake of giving their baby solid food when he is hungry, when what he really needs is an additional milk feed.

Babies should be given breast or infant formula milk for the whole of the first year. Ordinary cow's, goat's, or sheep's milk is not suitable as your baby's main drink, as it doesn't contain enough iron and other nutrients for proper growth. However, whole cow's milk can be used in cooking or with cereal when weaning. Dairy products like yogurt and cheese can be introduced once the first tastes of fruit and vegetables are accepted, and they are generally very popular with babies. Choose full-fat products as opposed to low-fat, as babies need the calories for proper growth.

Fresh is best

Fresh foods just do taste, smell, and look better than jars of pre-prepared baby foods. Nor is there any doubt that, prepared correctly, they are better for your baby (and you), for it is inevitable that nutrients, especially vitamins, are lost in the processing of pre-prepared baby foods. Homemade foods taste different from the jars you can buy. I believe your child will be less fussy and find the transition to joining in with family meals easier if he is used to a wide selection of fresh tastes and textures from an early age.

Organic

Organic fruit and vegetables are produced without artificial chemicals, such as pesticides and fertilizers. There is at present no scientific evidence that pesticide levels in ordinary foods are harmful to young babies and children, but some mothers prefer not to take the risk. It is an environmentally friendly option but it costs more, and it is up to you to decide whether it's worth the extra money.

GM foods

Genetic modification (GM) is the process of transferring genes from one species to another. For example, a tendency to resist damage from certain insects could be implanted from one plant to another. More research is needed to know whether genetically modified foods are of higher quality or whether the cost to humans and the environment outweighs any benefit.

Nutritional requirements

Proteins

Proteins are needed for the growth and repair of our bodies; any extra can be used to provide energy (or is deposited as fat). Proteins are made up of different amino acids. Some foods (meat, fish, soya beans, and dairy produce, including cheeses) contain all the amino acids that are essential to our bodies. Other foods (grains, legumes, nuts, and seeds) are valuable sources of protein but don't contain all the essential amino acids.

Carbohydrates

Carbohydrates and fat provide our bodies with their main source of energy. There are two types of carbohydrate: sugar and starch (which in complex form provides fiber). In both types there are two forms: natural and refined. The natural form provides a more healthy alternative.

Fats

Fats provide the most concentrated source of energy, and babies need proportionately more fat in their diet than adults. Energy-dense foods like cheese, meat, and eggs are needed to fuel their rapid growth and development, and fat provides more than 50 percent of the energy in breast milk. Foods that contain fats also contain fat-soluble vitamins A, D, E, and K, which are important for the healthy development of your baby. The problem is that many people eat too much fat and the wrong type.

There are two types of fat: 1) saturated (solid at room temperature), which mainly comes from animal sources and from artificially hardened fats found in cakes, cookies, and hard margarines, and 2) unsaturated (liquid at room temperature), which comes from vegetable sources. It is the saturated fats which are the most harmful and which may lead to high cholesterol levels and coronary disease later in life.

It is important to give your baby whole milk for at least the first two years, but try to reduce fats in cooking and use butter and margarine in moderation. Try to reduce saturated fats in your child's diet by cutting down on fatty meats like fatty ground meat or sausages and replace them with lean red meat, chicken, or oily fish.

Essential fatty acids (EFAs) are important for your baby's brain and visual development. There are two types of EFA – omega 6 from seed oils (e.g., sunflower, safflower, and corn) and omega 3 from oily fish (e.g., salmon, trout, sardines, and fresh tuna in moderation – not canned tuna). In general we get enough omega 6 in our diets; it is the omega 3 that is often low. The right balance of both types of EFAs is important, especially in early life.

Sugars
Natural
❀ Fruits and fruit juices
❀ Vegetables and vegetable juices
Refined
❀ Sugars and honey
❀ Sweetened drinks and soda
❀ Sweet gelatins
❀ Jellies and other preserves
❀ Cookies, cakes, and muffins

Starches
Natural
❀ Whole-grain breakfast cereals, flour, bread, and pasta
❀ Brown rice
❀ Potatoes
❀ Dried beans, lentils, peas, and other legumes
❀ Bananas and many other fruits and vegetables
Refined
❀ Processed breakfast cereals
   (e.g. sugar-coated flakes)
❀ White flour, breads, and pasta
❀ White rice
❀ Sugary cookies, cakes, and muffins

The essential vitamins and minerals

VITAMIN A
Essential for growth, healthy skin, tooth
enamel, and good vision. Also boosts
the immune system.
Liver
Oily fish
Carrots
Dark green leafy vegetables
(e.g. broccoli)
Orange and red fruit and vegetables
(e.g. carrots, red bell peppers, sweet potatoes,
tomatoes, apricots, mangoes, and squash)

VITAMIN B COMPLEX
Essential for growth, for changing food
into energy, for a healthy nervous system,
and as an aid to digestion. There are a
large number of vitamins in the B group.
Some are found in many foods, but no
foods except for liver and yeast extract
contain them all.
Meat
Sardines
Dairy produce and eggs
Whole-grain cereals
Dark green vegetables
Nuts
Legumes
Bananas

VITAMIN C
Needed for growth, healthy tissue,
and healing of wounds as it helps
to fight infection. It also helps in
the absorption of iron.
Vegetables such as:
broccoli, bell peppers, potatoes,
spinach and cauliflower
Fruits such as:
citrus fruits, blackcurrants, melon, papaya,
strawberries and kiwi fruit

VITAMIN D
Essential for proper bone formation,
it works in conjunction with calcium.
It's found in few foods, but is made
by the skin in the presence of sunlight.
Oily fish
Eggs
Margarine
Dairy produce

VITAMIN E
Important for the composition of the cell
structure. Helps the body create and
maintain red blood cells.
Vegetable oils
Avocados
Wheatgerm
Nuts and seeds

CALCIUM
Important for strong bones,
good teeth, and growth.
Dairy products
Canned fish with bones
(e.g. sardines)
Dried fruit
White bread
Green leafy vegetables
Legumes

IRON
Needed for healthy blood and muscles.
Iron deficiency is very common and will
leave your child feeling tired and run
down. Red meat is the best source of iron.
It's more difficult to absorb iron from
non-meat sources. However, if combined
with vitamin C-rich foods, iron absorption
can be increased by about 30 percent.
Red meat, especially liver
Oily fish
Egg yolks
Dried fruits (especially apricots)
Whole-grain and fortified cereals
Lentils and legumes
Green leafy vegetables

For most babies who eat fresh food in sufficient quantities and drink infant formula milk for the first year, vitamin supplements are probably unnecessary. If your baby is being breastfed, then vitamin D supplements may be needed after six months of age, as breast milk does not contain enough vitamin D. Your pediatrician will be able to advise you as to whether this is necessary.

Vegetarian families should speak to their pediatrician about an appropriate diet and also about vitamin and iron supplements. It is mainly vitamins A and D that are likely to be low in children aged six months to two years.

Vitamins are necessary for the correct development of the brain and nervous system. A good balanced diet should supply all the nutrients your child needs, and an excess of vitamins is potentially harmful, but children who are picky eaters could also benefit by taking a multivitamin supplement specially designed for children.

There are two types of vitamin – water-soluble (C and B complex) and fat-soluble (A, D, E, and K). Water-soluble vitamins cannot be stored by the body, so foods containing these should be eaten daily. They can also easily be destroyed by overcooking, especially when fruits and vegetables are boiled in water. You should try to preserve these vitamins by eating the foods raw or just lightly cooked (in a steamer, for instance).

High-risk foods
There are several food and dairy products that account for most food allergies (see the box on page 13). For normal healthy babies there is no evidence that starting solids later than age four to six months or delaying the introduction of potentially allergenic foods will affect the likelihood of developing allergies. In fact, feeding your baby a wide variety of foods, including the common food allergens such as eggs and fish, between six and nine months helps give your baby a wide repertoire of foods without increasing the chances of a food allergy developing.

If there is a history of food allergies in the family, or if your baby suffers from eczema, you will need to be more cautious when introducing new foods and consider introducing potentially allergenic foods one at a time to see if there is a reaction. If your baby has severe eczema, it may be worth having allergy testing done before you start solids to help pick up any allergies first. Studies have shown that children with severe eczema that started before six months are at particular risk of suffering a food allergy.

Food allergies can show up in two ways in babies. Immediate allergies result in rapid onset of itchy spots, swelling, and in rare severe cases, difficulty in breathing. Delayed allergies can show up with eczema, reflux, colic, or diarrhea, but food (most commonly milk) may be difficult to pin down as the cause due to delay in symptoms emerging. Redness caused by berries tends to happen only in kids with eczema. This is due to the irritating effect of the acid in the fruit, not an allergy, so you can let your baby eat them.

Potential high-risk foods
❀ Cow's milk and dairy products
❀ Nuts and seeds
❀ Eggs
❀ Wheat-based products
❀ Fish (especially shellfish)
❀ Chocolate

Water

Humans can survive for quite a time without food, but only a few days without water. Babies lose more water through their skin and kidneys than adults, and are particularly vulnerable to vomiting and diarrhea. Thus it's vital that they don't become dehydrated. Ensure your baby drinks plenty of fluids; cooled boiled water is the best drink to give on hot days – it's a better thirst quencher than any sugary beverage. Avoid bottled mineral water as it can contain high concentrations of mineral salts, which are unsuitable for babies.

It really isn't necessary to give a very young baby anything to drink other than milk or plain water if he is just thirsty. Fruit syrups, sodas, and sweetened herbal drinks should be discouraged, to prevent dental decay. Don't be fooled if the label says "dextrose" – this is just a type of sugar.

If your baby refuses to drink water, then give him fresh 100 percent fruit juice. Dilute according to instructions or use one part juice to three parts water.

The question of allergies

There is no need to worry unduly about food allergies unless you have a family history of allergies or atopic disease. The incidence of food allergies in babies with no family history of allergies is very small (approximately 6 percent).

Current advice is to breastfeed exclusively for four months and preferably six months, but solids can be introduced after four months (your pediatrician will advise on the right time to introduce solids to your baby) with no delay for allergenic foods. Some pediatricians suggest leaving two or three days between the introduction of each new food to check for allergic reactions, though delaying the introduction of foods does NOT reduce the incidence of food allergies. Don't remove key foods such as milk and wheat from your child's diet before consulting your pediatrician.

The good news is that children normally outgrow allergies to milk and eggs (around half by four to six years), but some allergies may last longer. Allergies to nuts, fish, and shellfish, however, are less commonly outgrown. Never be afraid to take your baby to the doctor if you are worried that something is wrong. Young babies' immune systems aren't fully matured and they can become ill very quickly and develop serious complications if they aren't treated properly.

Lactose intolerance

Hereditary lactose intolerance develops in late childhood and does not affect infants. Being born with complete lactose intolerance is beyond rare and some gastroenterologists suspect it doesn't actually exist.

The most common time you see lactose intolerance during infancy is when it occurs as the result of a tummy upset that causes swelling in the lining of the gut, temporarily reducing the amount of lactase enzyme in there. This causes diarrhea and bloating, but it lasts only for a few weeks. This is only temporary and should not be confused with cow's milk protein allergy. If your child is breastfed, continue, but if you are formula-feeding, he should change to a low-lactose formula for a few weeks, then back to normal formula. Soy milk doesn't contain lactose, but it is not recommended for babies under the age of six months due to the high levels of estrogen.

Lactose intolerance isn't actually an allergy, but rather the inability to digest lactose (the sugar in milk) because of a lack of a digestive enzyme. This is usually hereditary, particularly in darker-skinned people, and, if this is the case, your child may experience bloating, diarrhea, and gas, usually 30 minutes after having dairy foods. This means you should avoid giving foods containing large amounts of lactose, such as plain milk, cream, or soft cheeses.

Many cheeses and yogurts contain little lactose and so do not present a problem, but reduced-lactose milk products are widely available at the supermarket. Lactose intolerance that develops during later childhood will last for life.

Cow's milk protein allergy

In rare cases a baby may not be able to tolerate cow's milk protein, causing colic, sometimes bloody diarrhea, and a failure to thrive. In these cases you should seek the advice of your pediatrician on substitutes such as soy formulas, as some children who are allergic to cow's milk protein are also sensitive to soy protein and may need a more specialized formula.

Eggs

Babies can eat eggs from six months but eggs must be thoroughly cooked until both white and yolk are solid. Many people avoid giving yolk until one year, but there is no reason for this – you can give the whole egg.

Fruits

Some children have an adverse reaction to citrus or tomato. Allergies to tomato, citrus, and berries are very rare and the redness around the mouth is the irritant effect of fruit acid, most commonly noticed in children who already suffer from eczema. Occasionally, children can have an allergy to kiwifruit.

Honey

Honey should not be given to children under twelve months as it can cause infant botulism. Although this is very rare, it is best to be safe, as a baby's digestive system is too immature to deal with the bug.

Nuts

In the US it is estimated that just over 1 percent of children are allergic to peanuts. Peanuts and peanut products and tree nuts such as walnuts and hazelnuts can induce a severe allergic reaction (anaphylaxis), which can be life threatening, so it's best to be cautious if there is a history of allergy including hay fever, eczema, and asthma. If you are particularly concerned about nut allergies, for example if a sibling or parent suffers or there is a background of eczema, get your baby tested for allergies when you start weaning. For babies where there are no allergy concerns, peanut butter and finely ground nuts can be introduced from six months. However, whole and chopped nuts are not suitable before five years due to the risk of choking.

It used to be recommended that if there was a family history of peanut or nut allergies, mothers should avoid peanuts during pregnancy and breastfeeding and that the child should not have them for the first three years. However, advances in understanding have led to the withdrawal of this advice as avoiding peanuts does not appear to help reduce peanut allergy. If nuts are given after six months, they should be finely chopped. However, if there is particular concern about a nut allergy or a background of significant eczema, it would be advisable to have an allergy test done before introducing nuts.

Gluten

Gluten is found in wheat, rye, barley, and oats. Foods containing gluten, such as wheat-based cereals, bread, or tiny pasta shapes, can be introduced at six or seven months, ideally alongside breast milk.

When buying baby cereals, choose varieties that are gluten-free. Baby rice is the safest to try at first, and thereafter there are plenty of alternative gluten-free products such as soy, corn, rice, millet, rice noodles, and buckwheat spaghetti, and potato flours for thickening and baking.

In some cases, intolerance to wheat and similar proteins is temporary, and children may grow out of the condition before they are two or three years old. However, some people suffer from a permanent sensitivity to gluten known as celiac disease. Symptoms include loss of appetite, poor growth, swollen abdomen, and pale, particularly smelly stools. The disease can be diagnosed by a blood test.

Gastro-esophageal reflux disease (GERD)

GERD is caused when a weak valve at the top of the stomach allows the feed, along with gastric acid, to come back up, causing symptoms including vomiting and heartburn. All babies are born with this weak valve, but some regurgitate excessive amounts because of GERD. Regular vomiting, refusing feeds or managing only small amounts of milk at a time, losing or not gaining weight, or crying excessively after feeding can all be symptoms. If you are worried, take your baby to your pediatrician. GERD may also be caused by an underlying milk allergy, so if there is a family history of allergy and it gets worse when your child moves from breast to bottle or medication is ineffective, consult your pediatrician.

If your baby is diagnosed with GERD:
❀ Holding your baby in an upright position during and about 20 minutes after each feed can help.
❀ Your baby may sleep more comfortably if you raise the head of his bed so that he is sleeping on a slight incline. Keeping the upper part of the body elevated means gravity can help to keep his milk down.
❀ Try giving smaller, more frequent feeds.

❀ In more severe cases it can be worth trying feed thickeners (when breast- or bottle-feeding) but speak to your pediatrician for further advice. Your pediatrician may also prescribe a prethickened infant formula. Some babies also require antacid medicines. Most cases of GERD improve after starting solids, but for most babies this is not an indication to start solids early.

Preparing baby foods

Preparing and cooking baby foods isn't difficult, but because you're dealing with a baby, considerations like hygiene must be of the utmost importance. Always wash fruit and vegetables carefully before cooking.

Equipment

Most of the equipment you require will already be in your kitchen (for example, mashers, graters, and strainers), but the following four pieces may not be, and I consider them to be vital!

Food mill/baby food grinder. This hand-turned food mill, or ricer, purées the food, separating it from the seeds and tough fibers which can be difficult for the baby to digest. It is ideal for foods like dried apricots, corn, or green beans, and is also good for potato, which becomes sticky in a food processor or blender.

Electric hand blender/immersion blender. This is easy to clean and ideal for making small quantities of baby purées.

Blender or food processor. These are good for puréeing larger quantities when making batches for freezing.

Steamer. Steaming food is one of the best ways to preserve nutrients. It is worth buying a multi-tiered steamer, but a colander over a saucepan with a well-fitting lid is a cheaper alternative.

Sterilizing

At first, it is very important to sterilize bottles properly, and particularly the nipples, by whatever approved method you choose. Warm milk is the perfect breeding ground for bacteria, and if bottles are not properly washed and sterilized, your baby can become very ill. However, it is not necessary to sterilize the equipment you use for cooking, puréeing, or storing baby food, but take extra care to keep everything very clean.

Use a dishwasher if you have one, which helps to ensure the equipment is perfectly clean. Dry utensils with a clean dish towel or use paper towels.

Continue to sterilize all milk bottles and nipples until your baby is one year old. When your baby starts to crawl and put everything in reach into his mouth, there is really not much point sterilizing spoons or food containers. There is no need to sterilize other feeding equipment, but do wash bowls and spoons in a dishwasher or by hand in water that is as hot as you can handle wearing dishwashing gloves. If using a food mixer, rinse it out with boiling water, as mixers are a common breeding ground for germs.

Steaming

Steam the vegetables or fruits until tender. This is the best way to preserve the fresh taste and vitamins. Vitamins B and C are water-soluble and can easily be destroyed by overcooking, especially when foods are boiled in water. Broccoli loses over 60 percent of its antioxidants when boiled, but less than 7 percent when steamed.

Boiling

Peel, seed, or pit vegetables or fruits and cut up. Try to use only a little water and be careful not to overcook. To make a smooth purée, add just enough of the cooking liquid or a small amount of formula or breast milk.

Microwaving

Place the vegetables or fruit in a suitable dish. Add a little water, cover leaving an air vent, and cook on full power until tender (stir halfway through). Purée to the desired consistency. Check that it isn't too hot to serve to your baby and stir well to avoid hot spots.

Baking

If you are cooking a family meal in the oven, bake a potato, sweet potato, or butternut squash for your baby. Prick the vegetable and bake until tender. Cut in half (remove the seeds from the squash), scoop out the flesh, and mash with some water or milk.

Freezing baby foods

As a baby only eats tiny amounts, especially in the early stages of weaning, it saves time to make up larger quantities of purée and freeze extra portions in ice-cube trays or small plastic containers for future meals. This means that in a couple of hours you can prepare enough food for your baby for a month using the weekly menu planners (see pages 44–7).

Cook and purée the food, cover, and cool it as quickly as possible. To preserve quality, it is important that any foods to be frozen are covered. You can buy ice-cube trays made of a flexible material with lids. It is also best if the container is filled almost to the top, rather than leaving a pocket of air above the food. Food should be stored in a freezer that will freeze food to 0°F, or below, in 24 hours.

Once your baby starts eating larger portions, it is a good idea to buy some plastic containers with snap-on lids that are designed for freezing baby food. Always label frozen food with the contents and date you froze it. Thaw foods either by taking them out of the freezer several hours before a meal to thaw in the fridge, heating in a saucepan, or thawing in a microwave. Always reheat foods until piping hot, allow to cool, and always test the temperature of the food before giving it to your baby. If reheating in a microwave, make sure that you stir the food to get rid of any hot spots.

❀ Do not refreeze food that has previously been frozen. The exception to this is raw frozen food which can be cooked and then refrozen. For example, cooked frozen peas can be refrozen.

❀ Do not heat to thaw and then leave in the refrigerator to reheat and serve.

❀ If you have thawed baby food in the refrigerator overnight, it should be used within 24 hours. Once reheated, use within one hour as baby food is a prime breeding ground for bacteria.

❀ Sometimes you may need to add liquid when reheating frozen food as freezing can cause food to dry out.

❀ Baby foods can be stored in a freezer for up to eight weeks.

Introducing particular foods

In the box (opposite) I have listed particular foods you should avoid feeding your baby until a certain age. This is not an exhaustive list, and you should refer to each chapter and your pediatrician for more information.

Meal planners

In the next chapter I've devised meal planners to help you through the first weeks of introducing solids. The First Tastes Meal Planner (see pages 44–5) shows how to gradually introduce your baby to solids using mainly single ingredients such as easily digested fruit and vegetable purées that are unlikely to provoke an allergic reaction. Once your baby has been introduced to these tastes, progress to the After First Tastes Accepted Meal Planner (see pages 46–7), which includes combinations of fruit and vegetable purées like carrot and pea or peaches, apples, and pears. Adapt the recipes according to what is in season.

These planners are intended only as a guide and will depend on many factors including your baby's weight. If your baby's last meal is close to bedtime, avoid giving him anything that is heavy or difficult to digest. This is certainly not the time to experiment with new foods.

I have tried to give a wide choice of recipes, although I expect that, in practice, meals that your baby enjoys will be repeated several times – and this is where your freezer will come in handy.

In subsequent chapters, there are meal planners to follow or use as a guide. Adapt the charts according to what is in season and what you are preparing for your family. From nine months, you should be able to cook for your baby and family together, perhaps eating the recipes you give your baby for lunch and dinner for your own supper, provided you do not add salt to your baby's portion. Some babies may prefer four meals a day but, in these later charts, I have set out three meals which should be sufficient for most babies, especially with healthy snacks in between.

Many of the vegetable purées included in the early chapters can be transformed into a vegetable soup; and a number of the vegetable dishes can serve as good side dishes for the rest of the family. Again, if you give the baby some of the vegetables that you are preparing for the family, make sure they have not been salted. Many of the recipes in the later chapters are suitable for the whole family.

With each recipe are symbols of two faces – one smiling ☺, the other gloomy ☹. If you circle these, you will find them useful for recording your successes (or otherwise)! Some recipes also show a snowflake, which means the meal is suitable for freezing.

When can they have … ?
Gluten (wheat, rye, barley, and oats)
 6 months
Citrus fruits
 6 months
Well-cooked eggs
 6–9 months
Well-cooked scrambled eggs
 from 12 months
Added salt
 limited amount from 12 months
Sugar
 limited amount from 12 months
Whole cow's milk as a main drink
 12 months
Honey
 12 months
Paté
 12 months
Soft/blue cheese, e.g. Brie/Gorgonzola
 12 months
Whole/chopped nuts
 5 years

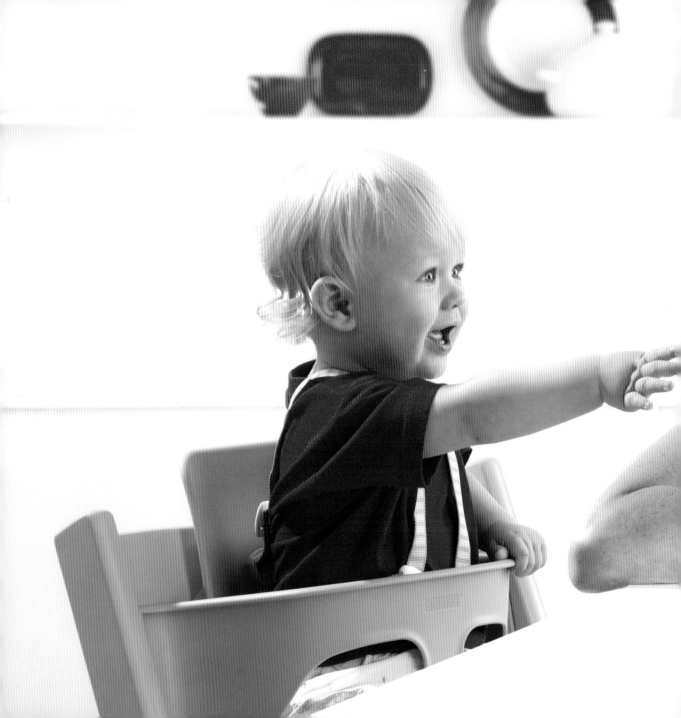

CHAPTER TWO
First-stage weaning

As discussed in chapter one, the US Department of Health and Human Services guidelines state that babies should be exclusively breastfed up to the age of six months. However, every baby is different, and signs that your baby could be ready to start solids are:

1 She is no longer satisfied by a full milk feed.
2 She is demanding increasingly frequent milk feeds.
3 She may start to wake in the night to feed after a period of sleeping through the night.
4 She is interested in watching others eat.
5 She is able to support her head and neck well when in a sitting position.

A baby's digestive system is not capable of absorbing foods more complex than baby milk before the age of at least 17 weeks. Always consult your pediatrician before commencing weaning.

Start by offering her very smooth, runny purées of apple, pear, carrot, sweet potato, potato, or butternut squash. You can also mix fruits and vegetables with baby rice. Don't expect your baby to eat much at all in the first week. Just offer solids once a day at first and choose a time when you are both relaxed and not in a hurry. She will need to be a little bit hungry but not ravenously so. You may need to give her a little milk to take the edge off her hunger first. Don't rush – try to go at your baby's pace.

A mother's instinct is very powerful, so if you feel she is ready, you are probably right. If she doesn't seem at all interested after a couple of attempts, you could always leave it another few days and then try again.

Also bear in mind that one of the reasons for the six-month recommendation is that breast milk is sterile, whereas, in underdeveloped countries, introducing solids early on can lead to infection.

First fruits and vegetables

Very first foods should be easy to digest and unlikely to provoke an allergic reaction. I find that root vegetables like carrot, sweet potato, parsnip, and rutabaga tend to be the most popular with very young babies due to their naturally sweet flavor and smooth texture once puréed. The best first fruits for young babies are apple, pear, banana, and papaya, but it's important that you choose fruit that is ripe and has a good flavor, so it's a good idea to taste it yourself before giving it to your baby.

Until recently, the advice given was to introduce each food separately, waiting for three days before introducing another new food. However, unless there is a history of allergy or you are concerned about your baby's reactions to a certain food, there is no reason why new foods should not be introduced on consecutive days, provided you keep to the list in the table (see page 24).

When introducing solids, take care not to reduce your baby's breast or infant formula milk intake, as milk is still the most important factor in growth and development.

It is important to wean your baby on as wide a range of foods as possible. After first tastes are accepted you can introduce all fruit and vegetables (see page 31). However, take care with citrus, pineapple, berry fruits and kiwi fruit as these may upset some susceptible babies.

Best first fruits	Best first vegetables
Apple	Carrot
Pear	Potato
Banana*	Rutabaga
Papaya*	Parsnip
	Pumpkin
	Butternut squash
	Sweet potato

Banana and papaya do not require cooking provided they are ripe. They can be puréed or mashed on their own or together with a little breast or infant formula milk. Bananas are not suitable for freezing.

Fruit

At first a baby should have cooked purées of fruits like apples and pears, or uncooked mashed banana or papaya. After the first few weeks your baby can graduate to other raw mashed or puréed fruits like melon, peach, and plum – these are delicious as long as they are ripe.

Dried fruits can be introduced but in small quantities; although they are nutritious they tend to be laxatives. If you are worried about the use of pesticides, organic fruit and vegetables are available.

Vegetables

Some people prefer to start their babies on vegetables rather than fruit in order to establish a liking for more savory tastes.

When introducing a baby to solids, it is best to start with root vegetables, particularly carrots, since they are naturally sweet. Different vegetables provide different vitamins and minerals (see chart on page 11) so a variety is of value at later stages.

Many vegetables have quite strong flavors – broccoli, for example – so when solids are fairly well established, you could mix in some potato or baby rice and milk to make it more palatable. Very young babies like their food quite bland.

Note that all fruit and vegetables can also be cooked in a microwave (see page 17 for method).

Rice

Another good first food is baby rice. Mixed with water or breast or infant formula milk, it is easily digested and its milky taste makes for a smooth transition to solids. Choose one that is sugar-free and enriched with vitamins and iron. Personally, I prefer to combine baby rice with fruit and vegetable purées.

Textures

At the very beginning of weaning, the rice and fruit or vegetable purées should be fairly wet and soft. This means that most vegetables, for instance, should be cooked until very soft so that they purée easily. You will probably need to thin out the consistency of the purées, since babies are more likely to accept food in a semi-liquid form. You can use infant formula or breast milk, fruit juice, or boiled water.

As your baby becomes more accustomed to the feel of "solid food" in her mouth, you can gradually start to reduce the amount of liquid that you are adding to the purées, which will encourage her to chew a little. This should be a natural process as she should want to chew her food as she starts teething (usually between six and twelve months). You could also thicken the purées if necessary with baby rice. As the baby becomes older and solid feeding is established (at the age of about six months), some fruit can be served raw and vegetables can be cooked more lightly (retaining more vitamin C).

Peel, core, and seed fruits as necessary before cooking and/or puréeing. Vegetables with fibers or seeds should be strained or put through a food mill for a smooth texture. The husks of legumes cannot be digested at this stage.

Quantities

At the very beginning, don't expect your baby to take more than 1–2 teaspoons of her baby rice or a fruit or vegetable purée. For this you should need one portion – in this section, this means one or two cubes from an ice-cube tray.

As your baby gets used to eating solids you may need to defrost three or more frozen food-cubes for her meal, or start freezing food in larger containers.

Drinks

Water is the best drink to offer. But freshly squeezed orange juice is high in vitamin C, which helps your child to absorb iron. If your baby reacts to orange juice, you can offer blackcurrant or rosehip instead. Dilute one part juice to at least five parts cooled boiled water. Diluted juice tastes weak to us but babies don't miss the sweet taste as they haven't been used to it. Try to avoid giving sweet drinks as this will give them a sweet tooth and result in them no longer accepting water.

If you buy commercial fruit juices, they should be unsweetened. But even those labeled "unsweetened" or "no added sugar" still contain sugars and acids that can lead to tooth decay. It is important not to let your baby continually sip any fluid except water.

A juicer is a useful appliance to have in the kitchen when there is a baby in the house. Many fruits and vegetables can be turned into nutritious drinks.

Tips for introducing solids

1 Make the rice or purée fairly wet and soft at first, using breast or infant formula milk, an unsweetened juice, or cooking water. A handy tip is to mix the purée in the plastic removable top of a feeding bottle (which has been sterilized).

2 Hold your baby comfortably on your lap or sit her in her baby chair. It would be better if both of you were protected against spills!

3 Choose a time when your baby is not frantically hungry and maybe give her some milk first to partially satisfy her – she will then be more receptive to the new idea.

4 Babies are unable to lick food off a spoon with their tongues, so choose a small, shallow plastic teaspoon off which she can take some food with her lips. (Special feeding spoons are available.)

5 Start by giving just one solid feed during the day, about 1–2 teaspoons to begin with. I prefer to give this feed at lunchtime.

Fruit and vegetables
FIRST TASTES

Apple
MAKES 5 PORTIONS
Choose a sweet variety of dessert apple. Peel, halve, core, and chop 2 medium apples. Put into a heavy saucepan with 4–5 tablespoons water. Cover and cook over a low heat until tender (7–8 minutes). Or steam for the same length of time. Purée. If steaming, add some of the boiled water from the bottom of the steamer to thin out the purée.

Apple and Cinnamon
Simmer 2 apples in apple juice or water with a cinnamon stick. Cook as above; remove stick before puréeing.

Pear
MAKES 5 PORTIONS
Peel, halve, and core 2 pears, then cut into small pieces. Cover with a little water, cook over a low heat until soft (about 4 minutes). Or steam for the same length of time. Purée. If the pears are very ripe, you may not need any water, and after the first few weeks of weaning, you can safely purée ripe pears without cooking. Apple and pear together make a good combination.

Banana

MAKES 1 PORTION

Mashed banana makes ideal baby food. It is easy to digest and rarely causes allergic reactions. Choose a ripe banana and mash very well with a fork to make it as smooth as possible. Add a little boiled water or breast or infant formula milk if it is too thick and sticky for your baby to swallow.

If your baby is suffering from diarrhea or a stomach upset, a diet of mashed banana, cooked apple purée, and baby rice for a few days is a good remedy.

Papaya

MAKES 4 PORTIONS

Papaya is an excellent fruit to give a very young baby. It has a pleasing sweet taste which is not too strong and blends within seconds to a perfect texture.

Cut a medium papaya in half, remove all the black seeds, and scoop out the flesh. Purée, adding a little breast or infant formula milk if you like.

Cream of Fruit

MAKES 3 EXTRA PORTIONS

Combining a fruit purée with breast or infant formula milk and baby rice can make it more palatable for your baby. In the next few months, when your baby may start eating some other exotic fruits like mango and kiwi fruit, this method of "diluting" the fruit purées with milk will also make them less acidic.

Peel, core, steam, or boil and purée the fruit as described and, for each 4-portion quantity of prepared fruit, stir in 1 tablespoon of unflavored baby rice or half a low-sugar rusk and 2 tablespoons of baby milk.

Three-Fruit Purée

MAKES 4 PORTIONS

This is a delicious combination of three of the first fruits that your baby can eat.

Mix 2 teaspoons each of pear and apple purées (see page 26) with half a banana, mashed. You could also use half a raw ripe pear, peeled, cored, and cut into chunks. Purée this and the half banana in a blender until smooth, then mix together with the 2 teaspoons of cooked apple purée.

Carrot or Parsnip

MAKES 4 PORTIONS

Peel, trim, and slice 2 medium carrots or parsnips. Place in a saucepan of lightly boiling water, cover, and simmer for 25 minutes or until very tender. Alternatively, you can steam them. Drain, reserving the cooking liquid, and purée to a smooth consistency, adding as much of the reserved liquid as necessary.

The cooking time is longer for small babies. Once your baby can chew, cut the cooking time down to preserve vitamin C and keep the vegetables crisper.

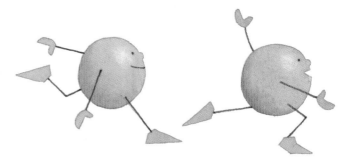

Sweet Potato, Rutabaga, or Parsnip

MAKES 4 PORTIONS

Use a large sweet potato, a small rutabaga or two large parsnips. Scrub, peel, and chop into small cubes. Cover with boiling water and simmer, covered, until tender (15–20 minutes). Alternatively, steam the vegetables. Drain, reserving the cooking liquid. Purée in a blender, adding some liquid if necessary.

Potato

MAKES 10 PORTIONS

Wash, peel, and chop 14 oz potatoes, just cover with boiling water and cook over a medium heat for about 15 minutes. Blend with some cooking liquid or breast or infant formula milk to make the desired consistency. Alternatively, steam the potatoes and blend with some water from the steamer or your baby's usual milk.

Avoid using a food processor or blender to purée potato as it breaks down the starch and makes a sticky pulp. Use a food mill instead.

You can bake potato or sweet potato in the oven. Preheat to 400°F for 1–1¼ hours or until soft. Scoop out the inside and mash with a little breast or infant formula milk and a pat of butter.

Cream of Carrot

MAKES 2 PORTIONS

A creamy purée can be made with many different vegetables by adding milk and baby rice. Make a purée with one large carrot (about 3 oz). This should make about ½ cup carrot purée (see page 28). Mix 1 tablespoon of unflavored baby rice with 2 tablespoons of your baby's usual milk. Stir the baby rice mixture into the vegetable purée.

Butternut Squash

MAKES 6 PORTIONS

Butternut squash is particularly good baked in the oven, as this caramelizes the natural sugars. Preheat the oven to 400°F. Cut a medium-sized butternut squash in half and remove the seeds and membranes. Place the halves cut side down on a well-oiled baking sheet lined with parchment paper and bake for about 45 minutes, or until the squash is tender. Remove from the oven, allow to cool, then scoop out the flesh and purée or mash with a little breast or formula milk or cooled boiled water. Alternatively, you can also peel and chop the squash and steam for about 20 minutes, until tender.

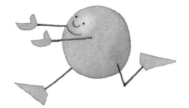

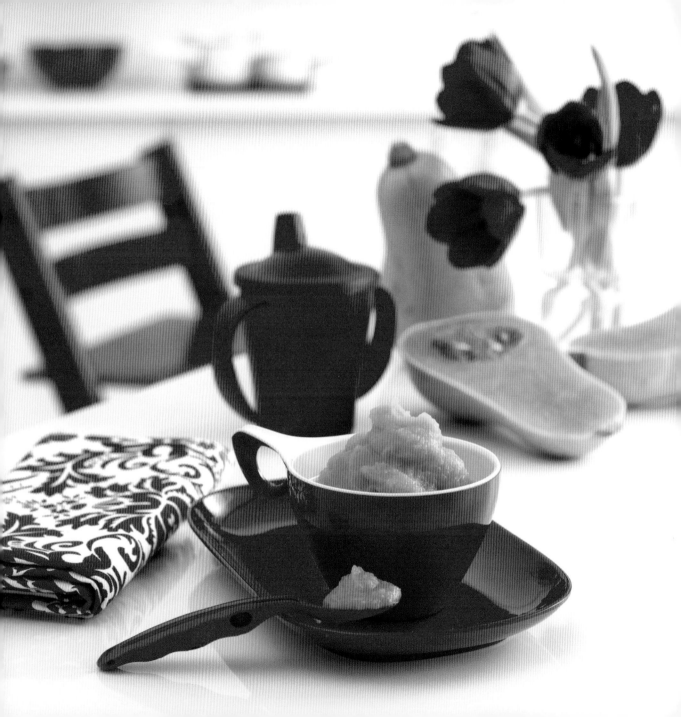

Fruit and vegetables
AFTER FIRST TASTES ACCEPTED

Zucchini
MAKES 8 PORTIONS

Wash 2 medium zucchini carefully, remove the ends, and slice. (The skin is soft so doesn't need to be removed.) Steam until tender (about 10 minutes), then purée in a blender or mash with a fork. (No need to add extra liquid.) Good mixed with sweet potato, carrot, or baby rice.

Broccoli and Cauliflower
MAKES 4 PORTIONS

Use 1 cup (about ¼ lb) of either. Wash well, cut into small florets, and add ⅔ cup boiling water. Simmer, covered, until tender (about 10 minutes). Strain, reserving the cooking liquid. Purée until smooth, adding a little of the liquid, or breast or infant formula milk, to make the desired consistency.

Alternatively, steam the florets for 10 minutes for better flavor and retention of nutrients. Add water from the steamer, or breast or infant formula milk, to make a smooth purée. Broccoli and cauliflower are good mixed with a cheese sauce or root vegetable purée like carrot or sweet potato.

Green Beans

Young green beans are best since they tend to be the least stringy variety. Wash the beans, top and tail, and remove any stringy bits. Steam until tender (about 12 minutes), then blend. Add a little boiled water or breast or infant formula milk to make a smooth purée. Green vegetables like beans are good mixed with root vegetables such as sweet potato or carrot.

Potato, Zucchini, and Broccoli
MAKES 4 PORTIONS

Combining potato with green vegetables makes them more palatable for babies. Peel and chop two medium potatoes (about ½ lb). Boil in water below a steamer for about 10 minutes or until soft. Place ¼ cup broccoli florets and ½ cup sliced zucchini in the steamer basket, cover and cook for 5 minutes or until all the vegetables are tender. Drain the potato and purée all the vegetables in a food mill, adding enough breast or infant formula milk to make a smooth consistency.

Broccoli Trio

MAKES 4 PORTIONS

Peel and chop a medium sweet potato (about ½ lb) and boil for 5 minutes. Place ½ cup each of broccoli and cauliflower florets in a steamer basket above the sweet potato, cover, and continue to cook for 5 minutes. When all the vegetables are tender, purée them in a blender together with a pat of butter and enough of the cooking liquid to make the desired consistency.

Carrot and Cauliflower

MAKES 4 PORTIONS

Combining vegetables makes them more interesting and, once your baby has got used to carrot and cauliflower separately, this combination makes a nice change. Cook ½ cup carrots, scraped and sliced, in boiling water for 20 minutes until soft. After 10 minutes, add 1½ cups cauliflower florets. Strain the vegetables and purée in a blender. Stir in 2 tablespoons of breast or infant formula milk.

Mango

MAKES 3 PORTIONS

Peel a ripe mango, removing the pit, and purée the flesh. No need to cook. Combines well with mashed banana.

Peach

MAKES 4 PORTIONS

Bring a small saucepan of water to the boil. Cut a shallow cross on the skin of 2 peaches, submerge them in the water for 1 minute, then plunge into cold water. Skin and chop the peaches, discarding the pits. Either purée the peaches uncooked or steam first for a few minutes until tender. Peach and banana makes a good combination.

Cantaloupe

MAKES 6 PORTIONS

Cantaloupes are the small, very pale green melons with orange flesh. They are rich in vitamins A and C. Only give ripe melon. Cut in half, remove seeds, scoop out the flesh, and purée in a blender.

Other varieties of sweet melon like Galia or honeydew are good too. When your baby is a little older, properly ripe melon may be eaten in pieces.

Plum

MAKES 4 PORTIONS

Skin 2 large ripe plums as for peaches (see above). Purée in a blender – the fruit can be puréed uncooked if soft and juicy or you could steam the plums for a few minutes until tender. Plums are good mixed with baby rice, banana, or yogurt.

Dried Apricot, Peach, or Prune

MAKES 4 PORTIONS

Many grocery stores stock a selection of ready-to-eat dried fruits. Dried apricots are particularly nutritious, being rich in betacarotene and iron. Avoid buying dried apricots that have been treated with sulphur dioxide – this preserves their bright orange color, but this substance can trigger asthma attacks in susceptible babies.

Cover 3/4 cup fruit with fresh cold water, bring to the boil, and simmer until soft (about 5 minutes). Drain, remove the pits, and press through a food mill to remove the rough skins. Add a little of the cooking liquid to make a smooth purée.

This is good combined with baby rice and milk, banana, or ripe pear.

Apricot and Pear

MAKES 8 PORTIONS

Roughly chop 1/2 cup ready-to-eat dried apricots and put them into a saucepan with 2 ripe Bosc pears (about 3/4 lb) peeled, cored, and cut into pieces. Cook, covered, over a low heat for 3–4 minutes. Purée in a blender. Alternatively, use 4 fresh, sweet, ripe apricots, peeled, pitted, and chopped.

Apple and Raisin Compote

MAKES 8 PORTIONS

Heat 3 tablespoons of fresh orange juice in a saucepan. Add 2 dessert apples peeled, cored, and sliced, and 2 tablespoons of washed raisins. Cook gently for about 5 minutes until soft, adding a little water if necessary.

Dried fruit like apricots or raisins should be put through a food mill for young babies, to get rid of the outer skin which is difficult to digest.

Peas

MAKES 4 PORTIONS

I tend to use frozen peas as they are just as nutritious as fresh. Cover 1 cup peas with water, bring to the boil and simmer, covered, for 4 minutes until tender. Strain, reserving some cooking liquid. Purée using a food mill or press through a strainer and add some of the cooking liquid to make the desired consistency. Good combined with potato, sweet potato, parsnip, or carrot. If using fresh peas, cook them for 12–15 minutes.

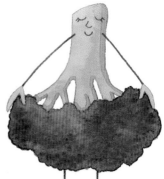

Red Bell Pepper

MAKES 2–3 PORTIONS

Wash, core, and seed a medium red bell pepper. Cut into quarters and roast under a preheated broiler until the skin is charred. Place in a plastic bag and let cool. Peel off the blistered skin and purée. Good with cauliflower, sweet potato, or potato.

Avocado

MAKES 1 PORTION

Cut a well-ripened avocado in half and scoop out the stone. Use ⅓–½ and mash the flesh with a fork, maybe adding a little milk. Serve quickly to avoid it turning brown. Good mixed with mashed banana.

Do not freeze avocados.

Corn on the Cob

MAKES 2 PORTIONS

Remove and discard the outer corn husks and silk from the corn and rinse well. Cover with boiling water and cook over a medium heat for 10 minutes. Strain and then cut off the kernels of corn using a sharp knife. Purée in a food mill. Alternatively, cook some frozen corn and then purée.

Spinach

MAKES 2 PORTIONS

Wash 2 cups spinach leaves very carefully, removing the coarse stalks. Either steam the spinach or put in a saucepan and sprinkle with a little water. Cook until the leaves are wilted (about 3–4 minutes). Gently press out any excess water. Good combined with potato, sweet potato, or butternut squash.

Tomatoes

MAKES 2–3 PORTIONS

Plunge 2 medium tomatoes in boiling water for 30 seconds. Transfer to cold water, skin, seed, and roughly chop. Melt a pat of butter in a heavy-bottomed saucepan and sauté the tomato until mushy. Purée in a blender. This is good combined with potato, cauliflower, or zucchini.

Peach and Banana ☺☹

This is a delicious purée to make when peaches are in season. They are a good source of vitamin C and are easy to digest. Banana also combines well with papaya.

MAKES 1 PORTION

1 ripe peach, skinned, pitted, and cut into pieces
1 small banana, peeled and sliced
½ tablespoon pure apple juice
baby rice (optional)

Put the peach, banana, and apple juice into a small pan, cover and simmer for 2–3 minutes. Purée in a blender. If it's too runny, add a little baby rice.

Three-Fruit Purée ☺☹

This makes a nice change from plain mashed banana or apple purée. When your baby is six months or older, you can make this with raw grated apple and mashed banana.

MAKES 1 PORTION

¼ dessert apple, peeled, cored, and chopped
¼ banana, peeled and chopped
1 teaspoon orange juice

Steam the apple until tender (about 7 minutes), then purée or mash it together with the banana and orange juice. Serve as soon as possible.

Peaches, Apples, and Pears ❄ ☺ ☹

When peaches aren't in season you can make this just using apples and pears.
If the purée is too thin, stir in some baby rice to thicken it.

MAKES 8 PORTIONS
2 dessert apples, peeled, cored, and chopped
1 vanilla bean
2 tablespoons apple juice or water
2 ripe peaches, skinned, pitted, and chopped
2 ripe pears, peeled, cored, and chopped

Put the chopped apple in a saucepan. Split the vanilla bean with a sharp knife,
scrape the seeds into the pan, and add the vanilla bean and apple juice or water.
Simmer, covered, for about 5 minutes. Add the peaches and pears and cook for
3–4 minutes more. Remove the vanilla bean and purée.

Mixed-Dried-Fruit Compote ❄ ☺ ☹

Dried fruit concentrates the goodness of the original fruit. Dried apricots and
prunes are a good source of iron and dried apricots are also rich in betacarotene.
Their natural sweetness makes them good first foods and I like to mix them with
fresh fruit. Prunes are a well-known laxative, so they are good mixed with apple
or pear if your baby is constipated.

MAKES 6 PORTIONS
½ cup each dried apricots, dried peaches, and prunes, roughly chopped
1 dessert apple and 1 pear, peeled, cored, and chopped, or 1 apple
   and 3 fresh apricots, skinned, pitted, and chopped

Put the dried fruit, apple, and pear (or apricot, if using) into a saucepan and just
cover with boiling water. Simmer for about 8 minutes. Strain the fruit and purée,
adding a little of the cooking liquid if necessary.

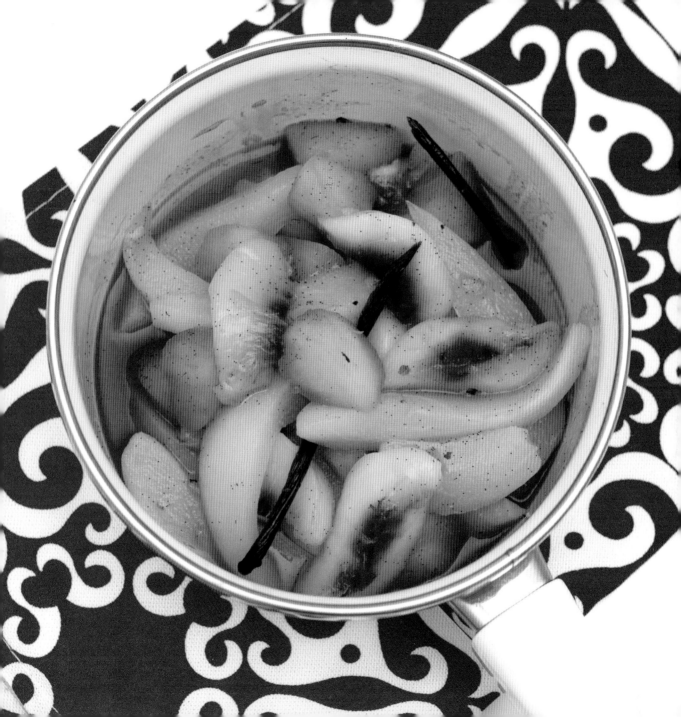

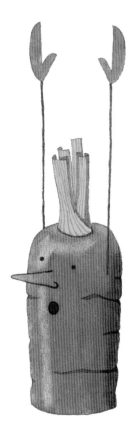

Vegetable Broth ❄ ☺ ☹

Vegetable broth forms the basis of many vegetable recipes. This should keep for a week in the refrigerator and it is well worth making your own, which will be free from additives and salt.

MAKES ABOUT 3³/4 CUPS
1 large onion, peeled
1 large carrot (about 5 oz), peeled
1 celery stick
1¹/2 cups mixed root vegetables (sweet potato,
    swede, parsnip), peeled and roughly chopped
¹/2 leek
2 tablespoons butter
1 bouquet garni
1 sprig of fresh parsley
1 bay leaf
6 black peppercorns
1¹/2 quarts water

Melt the butter in a large saucepan and sauté the onion for 5 minutes. Add the remaining ingredients and cover with the water. Bring to a boil and simmer for about 1 hour. Strain the broth and squeeze any remaining juices from the vegetables through a strainer.

Carrot and Pea Purée ☺ ☹

Both carrots and peas have a naturally sweet taste that appeals to babies.

MAKES 2 PORTIONS
2 medium carrots (about 7 oz), peeled and sliced
¹/3 cup frozen peas

Put the sliced carrots in a saucepan and cover with boiling water. Cook, covered, for 15 minutes. Add the peas and cook for a further 5 minutes. Purée with sufficient cooking liquid to make a smooth purée.

Trio of Vegetables ❄ ☺ ☹

When introducing green vegetables like broccoli, it's a good idea to combine them with sweet-tasting root vegetables such as sweet potato. If possible, it's a good idea to use a multi-layered steamer to prepare the vegetables.

MAKES 4 PORTIONS
1⅔ cups peeled and roughly chopped sweet potato
1 teaspoon vegetable or canola oil
3 tablespoons finely chopped onion
½ cup small broccoli florets
¼ cup frozen peas
½ cup vegetable broth (see opposite) or water

Steam the sweet potato for 6 minutes. Meanwhile, sauté the onion in the oil for about 5 minutes, until softened. Add the broccoli to the steamer and steam for 4 minutes, then add the peas and steam for 2–3 minutes. Mix the sautéed onion with the sweet potato, broccoli, and peas and add the vegetable broth or water from the steamer. Blend to make a purée. Add more liquid, if necessary, to make a smooth consistency.

Sweet Vegetable Medley ❄ ☺ ☹

Root vegetables like rutabaga, carrot, and parsnip make delicious and nutritious purées for young babies. You could also use butternut squash and pumpkin.

MAKES 5 PORTIONS
1 cup carrot, peeled and chopped
1 cup rutabaga, peeled and chopped
1 cup potato, butternut squash or pumpkin, peeled and chopped
½ cup parsnip, peeled and chopped
1¼ cups water or milk (can use cow's milk in cooking from six months)

Put the vegetables in a saucepan with the water or milk. Bring to a boil, then cover and simmer for 25–30 minutes or until the vegetables are tender. Remove with a slotted spoon and purée the vegetables in a blender, together with as much cooking liquid as necessary to make the desired consistency.

Watercress, Potato, and Zucchini Purée ❄ ☺ ☹

Watercress is rich in calcium and iron. It blends well with the other vegetables to make a tasty, bright green purée. You can add a little milk if your baby prefers it that way.

MAKES 6 PORTIONS
1 large potato (about 11 oz), peeled and chopped
1¼ cups vegetable broth (see page 38)
1 medium zucchini (about ¼ lb), trimmed and sliced
a small bunch of watercress
a little milk (optional)

Put the potato into a saucepan, cover with the broth, and cook for 5 minutes. Add the sliced zucchini and continue to cook for another 5 minutes. Trim the stalks of the watercress, add to the potato, and cook for 2–3 minutes. Purée the mixture in a food mill and, if you like, add a little milk to adjust the consistency.

Avocado and Banana or Papaya ☺ ☹

This is very simple to make and the fruits blend well. Babies need nutrient-dense foods to fuel their rapid growth and avocados are ideal because they contain more nutrients than any other fruit.

MAKES 1 PORTION
½ small avocado
½ small banana or ¼ papaya

Remove the flesh from the avocado and mash with the banana or papaya until smooth. This should be eaten soon after it is made or the avocado will turn brown.

Sweet Potato and Squash Purée ✳ ☺ ☹

Baking sweet potato and squash in a foil package intensifies the flavor and helps to retain vitamins. Add a little ground cinnamon if you like.

MAKES 5 PORTIONS
1 small or ½ large butternut squash, peeled, seeded, and cut into 1-inch cubes
1 sweet potato, peeled and cut into 1-inch cubes
a generous pat of butter
2 tablespoons water
a little breast or formula milk

Preheat the oven to 400°F. Lay a large piece of aluminum foil on a baking sheet and spread out the squash and sweet potato. Melt the butter, brush it over the vegetables, and sprinkle them with the water. Cover with a second piece of foil and scrunch the edges together to form a package. Bake for 30 minutes or until the vegetables are tender. Cool them slightly, then transfer to a blender (with any liquid in the bottom of the package). Blend to a smooth purée. If necessary, thin it with a little milk.

Squash and Pear Purée variation. Peel and chop 1 medium butternut squash and steam for 12 minutes. Peel, core, and chop 1 ripe pear, add to the steamer, and cook for 5 minutes or until the squash is tender. Purée in a blender.

Baked Sweet Potato ✳ ☺ ☹

Baking a sweet potato caramelizes the natural sugars, giving it a rich flavor.

MAKES 4 PORTIONS
1 large or 2 medium sweet potatoes

Preheat the oven to 400°F. Pierce each potato several times with a fork. Bake for about 1 hour, depending on their size. Remove from the oven and set aside until cool enough to handle. The skins should peel off easily. Cut the flesh into chunks and purée until smooth, adding a little breast or formula milk, or cooled boiled water, 1 tablespoon at a time, until you reach the desired consistency. If you like, you can mix the baked sweet potato flesh with apple purée or add a little ground cinnamon.

Leek, Sweet Potato, and Pea Purée ❄ ☺ ☹

Sweet potatoes make perfect baby food; they are full of nutrients and have a naturally sweet taste and smooth texture. Choose the orange-fleshed variety as it is rich in beta carotene. It is fine to use frozen vegetables in baby purées as they are frozen within hours of being picked and can be just as nutritious as fresh vegetables. Once cooked, frozen vegetables can be refrozen.

MAKES 5 PORTIONS
³/₄ cup leek, thoroughly washed and sliced
3¹/₂ cups sweet potato, peeled and chopped
1¹/₄ cups vegetable broth (see page 38)
¹/₂ cup frozen peas

Put the leek and sweet potato in a saucepan, pour over the vegetable broth, and bring to a boil. Cover and simmer for 15 minutes. Add the peas and continue to cook for 5 minutes. Purée in a blender.

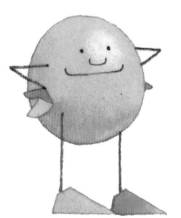

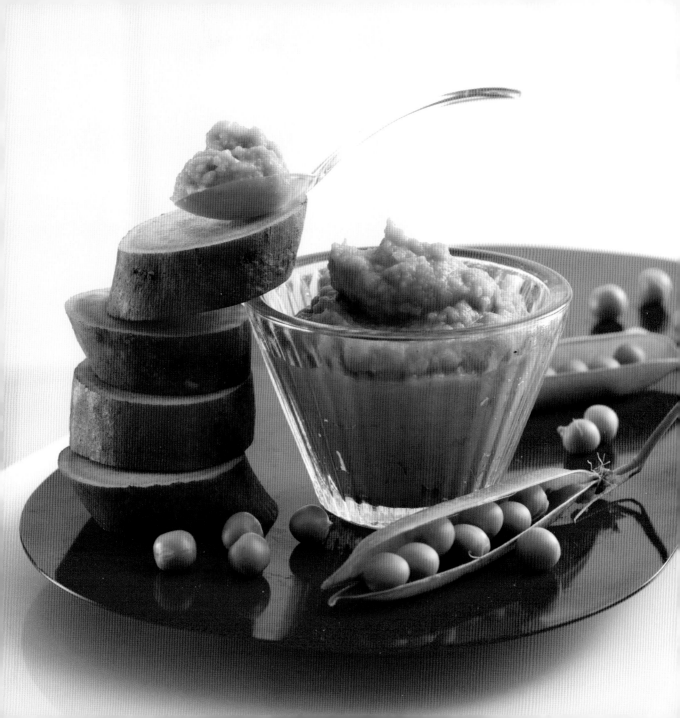

First tastes meal planner

Week 1	Early morning	Breakfast	Lunch	Dinner	Bedtime
Days 1–2	Breast/bottle	Breast/bottle	Breast/bottle Baby rice	Breast/bottle	Breast/bottle
Days 3–4	Breast/bottle	Breast/bottle	Breast/bottle Root vegetable e.g. carrot or sweet potato	Breast/bottle	Breast/bottle
Day 5	Breast/bottle	Breast/bottle	Breast/bottle Pear with baby rice	Breast/bottle	Breast/bottle
Day 6	Breast/bottle	Breast/bottle	Breast/bottle Apple	Breast/bottle	Breast/bottle
Day 7	Breast/bottle	Breast/bottle	Breast/bottle Vegetable e.g. butternut squash or sweet potato	Breast/bottle	Breast/bottle
Week 2					
Days 1–2	Breast/bottle Apple or pear with baby rice	Breast/bottle	Breast/bottle Root vegetable e.g. potato, parsnip, or carrot	Breast/bottle	Breast/bottle
Days 3–4	Breast/bottle Banana or papaya	Breast/bottle	Breast/bottle **Sweet Vegetable Medley**	Breast/bottle	Breast/bottle
Days 5–6	Breast/bottle Apple or pear	Breast/bottle	Breast/bottle Sweet potato, butternut squash, or rutabaga	Breast/bottle	Breast/bottle
Day 7	Breast/bottle Peach and banana or mashed banana	Breast/bottle	Breast/bottle Carrot or carrot and parsnip	Breast/bottle	Breast/bottle

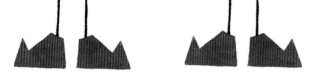

Week 3	Early morning	Breakfast	Lunch	Dinner	Bedtime
Day 1	Breast/bottle	Breast/bottle Banana	Diluted juice or water **Sweet Vegetable Medley**	Breast/bottle	Breast/bottle
Day 2	Breast/bottle	Breast/bottle Apple	Diluted juice or water **Sweet Vegetable Medley**	Breast/bottle	Breast/bottle
Day 3	Breast/bottle	Breast/bottle **Peaches, Apples, and Pears**	Diluted juice or water **Broccoli Trio**	Breast/bottle	Breast/bottle
Day 4	Breast/bottle	Breast/bottle **Cream of Fruit**	Diluted juice or water **Sweet Potato and Squash Purée**	Breast/bottle	Breast/bottle
Day 5	Breast/bottle	Breast/bottle **Cream of Fruit**	Diluted juice or water **Sweet Potato and Squash Purée**	Breast/bottle	Breast/bottle
Day 6	Breast/bottle	Breast/bottle Banana or papaya	Diluted juice or water **Potato, Zucchini, and Broccoli**	Breast/bottle	Breast/bottle
Day 7	Breast/bottle	Breast/bottle Pear or baby rice	Diluted juice or water **Carrot and Pea Purée**	Breast/bottle	Breast/bottle

These charts are intended only as a guide and will depend on many factors including your baby's weight. Some babies may want only one solid feed a day and some may prefer to have a second meal at dinnertime. Bold type indicates recipes shown in the book.

Fruit juice should be diluted at least three parts water to one part juice, or replaced completely with cooled boiled water.

After first tastes accepted meal planner

	Early morning	Breakfast	Lunch	Dinner	Bedtime
Day 1	Breast/bottle	Breast/bottle **Three-Fruit Purée**	**Leek, Sweet Potato, and Pea Purée** Breast/bottle	**Carrot and Cauliflower** Diluted juice or water	Breast/bottle
Day 2	Breast/bottle	Breast/bottle **Three-Fruit Purée**	**Leek, Sweet Potato, and Pea Purée** Breast/bottle	**Sweet Vegetable Medley** Diluted juice or water	Breast/bottle
Day 3	Breast/bottle	Breast/bottle Pear and baby cereal	**Broccoli Trio** Breast/bottle	Sweet potato Diluted juice or water	Breast/bottle
Day 4	Breast/bottle	Breast/bottle **Apple and Cinnamon**	**Trio of Vegetables** Breast/bottle	Sweet potato Diluted juice or water	Breast/bottle
Day 5	Breast/bottle	Breast/bottle Mango and baby cereal	**Avocado and Banana** Breast/bottle	**Carrot and Pea Purée** Diluted juice or water	Breast/bottle
Day 6	Breast/bottle	Breast/bottle Banana	**Watercress, Potato, and Zucchini Purée** Breast/bottle	**Broccoli Trio** Diluted juice or water	Breast/bottle
Day 7	Breast/bottle	Breast/bottle **Apple and Banana with Orange Juice**	**Watercress, Potato, and Zucchini Purée** Breast/bottle	**Broccoli Trio** Diluted juice or water	Breast/bottle

These charts are intended only as a guide and will depend on many factors including your baby's weight. Some babies will manage to eat some fruit after lunch and dinner.

* Fruit juice should be diluted at least three parts water to one part juice, or replaced completely with cooled boiled water.

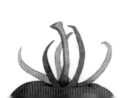
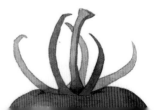

	Breakfast	Mid-morning	Lunch	Mid-afternoon	Dinner	Bedtime
Day 1	Breast/bottle Baby cereal Mashed banana	Breast/bottle	**Leek, Sweet Potato, and Pea Purée** Water or juice*	Breast/bottle	Carrot, mango, or peach; Yogurt Diluted juice or water	Breast/bottle
Day 2	Breast/bottle Baby cereal **Apple and Raisin Compote**	Breast/bottle	**Avocado and Banana** Diluted juice or water	Breast/bottle	**Carrot and Pea Purée** Cantaloupe melon Water or juice*	Breast/bottle
Day 3	Breast/bottle Baby cereal Mango and banana	Breast/bottle	**Baked Sweet Potato** Diluted juice or water	Breast/bottle	**Potato, Zucchini, and Broccoli** Yogurt Diluted juice or water	Breast/bottle
Day 4	Breast/bottle Baby cereal Yogurt	Breast/bottle	**Broccoli Trio** Diluted juice or water	Breast/bottle	**Sweet Vegetable Medley** Mango or papaya Water or juice*	Breast/bottle
Day 5	Breast/bottle Baby cereal **Peaches, Apples, and Pears**	Breast/bottle	**Broccoli Trio** Diluted juice or water	Breast/bottle	**Sweet Vegetable Medley** Sticks of toast Yogurt Water or juice*	Breast/bottle
Day 6	Breast/bottle Baby cereal **Peaches, Apples, and Pears**	Breast/bottle	**Watercress, Potato, and Zucchini Purée** Diluted juice or water	Breast/bottle	**Leek, Sweet Potato, and Pea Purée** Banana Water or juice*	Breast/bottle
Day 7	Breast/bottle Baby cereal **Apricot and Pear**	Breast/bottle	**Carrot and Pea Purée** Diluted juice or water	Breast/bottle	**Watercress, Potato, and Zucchini Purée** **Peach and Banana** Water or juice*	Breast/bottle

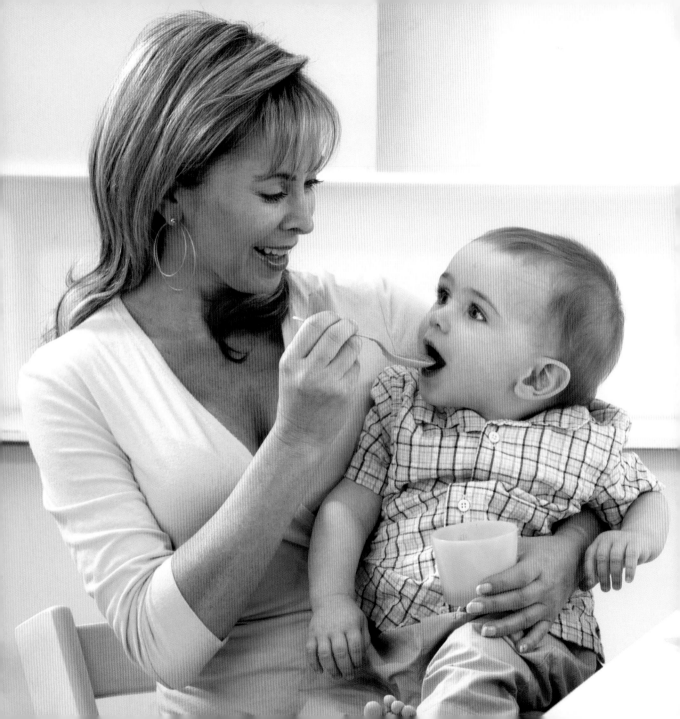

CHAPTER THREE

Second-stage weaning

Between seven and nine months is a rapid development period for your baby. A seven-month-old baby still needs to be supported whilst you are feeding him and, more often than not, still has no teeth. A nine-month-old baby, however, is usually strong enough to sit in a highchair whilst he is being fed and has already cut a few teeth. Babies of eight months are usually quite good at holding food themselves and enjoy eating small finger foods like cooked pasta, pieces of raw or cooked vegetables, or raw fruits. (Turn to pages 95–7 for suitable finger foods for young babies.) Babies are born with a store of iron that lasts for about six months. After this they rely on their diet for the iron they need. If a baby doesn't have at least 18 oz (2¼ cups) breast milk or infant formula per day, his daily intake of iron is likely to be below the recommended level, and this can impair his mental and physical development. It is particularly important not to use ordinary cow's milk for your baby's regular drink before the age of one year as it doesn't contain as much iron or vitamins as infant formula milk.

Less milk, more appetite

Once your baby is seven to eight months old, you can start cutting down on his milk so that he is more hungry for his solids. However, between six months and one year, babies should have 18–21 oz (2¼–2½ cups) breast milk or infant formula per day. In addition you can give other dairy products and offer water, diluted fruit juice or low-sugar herbal beverages with meals if your baby seems thirsty.

It is best to put only infant formula, breast milk, or water into your baby's bottle. Comfort-sucking on sweetened beverages is the main cause of tooth decay in young children, and babies are more vulnerable to decay than children or adults. You should start using a lidded cup with a soft spout and easy-to-hold handles once your baby is six months old. There are training cups available to guide your baby from a soft spout to open drinking cup in easy stages.

Let your baby's appetite determine how much he eats and never force him to eat something he actually dislikes. Don't offer it for a while, but reintroduce it a few weeks later. You may find that second time around he loves it.

Remember, at this age it is normal for babies to be quite chubby. As soon as your baby starts crawling and walking, he will lose this excess weight.

For those babies who dislike milk and are drinking less than 21 oz (2½ cups), use milk in recipes like Cauliflower Cheese (page 67). Also a small children's-size pot of yogurt or a matchbox-size piece of cheese is equivalent to 2 oz (¼ cup) milk.

Although a low-fat diet is fine for adults, it is not appropriate for young children, who need calories to grow. Give whole milk and avoid low-fat dairy products in the first two years.

The foods to choose

Your baby can now eat protein foods like eggs, cheese, legumes, chicken, and fish. Limit some foods which might be indigestible – such as spinach, lentils, cheese, or berry or citrus fruit – and don't worry if some foods, like legumes, peas, and raisins, pass through your child undigested: until they are about two years old, babies cannot completely digest husked vegetables and the skins of fruits. Peeling, mashing, and puréeing fruit and vegetables will of course aid digestion. With foods like bread, flour, pasta, and rice, try to choose whole-grain, rather than refined, as it is more nutritious.

Once your baby has passed the six-month stage and is happily eating bread and other foods containing gluten, there is no longer any need to give him special baby cereals. You can use adult cereals like instant oatmeal Cheerios, and graham crackers, which are just as nutritious and much cheaper. Choose a cereal that isn't highly refined and which is low in sugar and salt. Many people continue to use commercial baby foods because they think, due to the long list of vitamins and minerals on the packet, that they are more nutritious. However, babies who eat a good balanced diet of fresh foods get a perfectly adequate quantity of vitamins and minerals. Also, baby foods in general are heavily processed, and their finer texture and bland flavors will hinder the development of your baby's tastes.

Beware, too, of some of the teething biscuits you can buy which are supposedly the "ideal food for your baby." Many are full of sugar (some contain more sugar than a doughnut). Give your baby some toast to chew on or follow the simple recipe for teething biscuits in the nine-to-twelve-month finger food section (see page 97).

Ordinary cow's milk isn't suitable as your baby's main drink for the first year, as it doesn't contain enough iron or other nutrients for proper growth. However, whole cow's milk can be used in cooking or with cereal.

It is very difficult to give portion sizes as the quantities that babies eat vary enormously. The amount of food one baby needs to eat to maintain the same growth rate can be very different to the next baby, even if they are the same age and weight. They have different metabolic rates and different activity levels, and the food that their parents make can vary in calorie content significantly. The amount a baby eats can also vary from week to week and this is perfectly normal. By seven months, babies should ideally be having three solid meals a day. It's a good idea to take your child to be weighed regularly by your pediatrician. If he is growing along one percentile line on his growth chart and not crossing up or down lines, then he is eating the right amount – this is because babies can drop a couple of lines then grow along a lower one, leading to abnormal growth and failure to fulfil their genetic potential.

Fruit

Your baby should now be able to eat all fruits, and both fresh and dried fruits make a great snack. Different fruits contain different vitamins, so include as much variety as possible. Dried fruits are also a good source of other nutrients and energy, but need to be chopped into small pieces to reduce the risk of choking. Take care to remove any pits before giving fruit, and don't give whole grapes to young babies as they may choke on them.

Vitamin C boosts iron absorption so it's important to include vitamin C-rich fruits like citrus or berry fruits in your child's diet. It's good to give cereal with diluted orange juice in the morning. Orange juice also combines well with savory foods like carrot, fish, and liver. To begin with, give berry and citrus fruits in small quantities as they can be indigestible, and some babies can have an adverse reaction to them. Combine them with other fruits like apple, banana, pear, or peach. Kiwi fruit can also cause an allergic reaction in some young children. This is rare, but do watch your baby closely, especially if there is a family history of allergies or conditions such as eczema or asthma.

Vegetables

Your baby is now able to eat all vegetables, but if certain flavors – like that of spinach or broccoli – are too strong, try mixing them together with a cheese sauce or with root vegetables like sweet potato, carrot, or potato. Combinations of vegetables and fruit are also good – try butternut squash and apple, or spinach and pear. Steamed vegetables, like carrot sticks or small florets of cauliflower, make good finger food.

Frozen vegetables are frozen within hours of being picked, thus sealing in all the nutrients, so it's absolutely fine to use them to make your baby's purées. Whilst you cannot thaw and refreeze frozen foods, e.g. baby purées, this does not apply to frozen vegetables; you can use these to make baby purées and then refreeze them.

Eggs

Eggs are an excellent source of protein and also contain iron and zinc. They can be given from six months, but don't serve raw or lightly cooked eggs

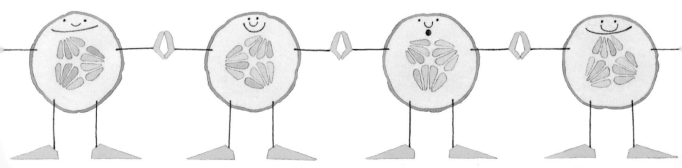

to babies under one year as there is a risk of salmonella. The white and yolk should be cooked until solid. Hard-boiled eggs, omelets, and well-cooked scrambled eggs are quick to cook and nutritious.

A vegetarian diet

A vegetarian diet can be fine for babies and small children as long as it is carefully balanced and does not contain too much fiber. Unlike adults, a bulky high-fiber diet is unsuitable for children as it is too low in calories and essential fats and hinders their absorption of iron. The nutrients that you will need to pay extra attention to are protein, iron, zinc, and the B vitamins – these are usually provided by meat. Below is a list of foods that you should include in a vegetarian baby's diet:

Dairy products, eggs, beans, lentils, fortified breakfast cereals, legumes (e.g. lentils), soya (e.g. tofu), green vegetables (e.g. spinach and broccoli), dried fruit

Fish

Many children grow up disliking fish as they find it bland and boring, so I try to mix it with stronger tastes, like salmon with carrots, tomato, and grated Cheddar or my tasty combination of fillets of cod with grated cheese, orange juice, and crushed cornflakes (believe me, it's yummy). If your child gets excited at the prospect of fish for dinner, then you deserve to be a very proud parent indeed.

If fish is overcooked, it becomes tough and tasteless. It is cooked when it just flakes with a fork but is still firm. Always check very carefully for bones before serving.

It's hard to find jars of purée containing fish; however, oily fish like salmon, trout, fresh tuna, and sardines are particularly important for the development of a baby's brain, nervous system, and vision and ideally should be included in the diet twice a week. Fats are a major component of the brain – for this reason, 50 percent of the calories of breast milk are composed of fat.

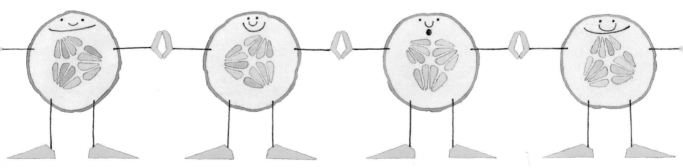

Meat

Chicken is an ideal first meat. It blends well with root vegetables like carrot and sweet potato, which give chicken purée a smoother texture. Chicken also works well with fruits like apple and grape. Homemade chicken broth forms the basis of many recipes so I recommend that you make large batches. It will keep in the fridge for 3–4 days. However, do not use frozen broth to make purées and then refreeze it. You can buy unsalted, ready-made broth.

As well as chicken breast, try also using the thigh meat – the dark meat of chicken contains twice as much iron and zinc as the white.

Iron deficiency anemia is the most common nutritional problem during early childhood, the symptoms of which can be hard to detect: your baby may just be tired and pale and more prone to infection, or his growth and development may seem to slow down. Red meat provides the best source of iron, particularly liver, which is ideal for babies as it has a soft texture and is easy to digest. Babies often reject red meats, not because of the taste but the chewy texture. It's a good idea to combine it with root vegetables or pasta, as they help to produce a texture that is much smoother and easier to swallow.

Iron is important for your baby's brain development, especially between six months and two years. The iron a baby inherits from his mother runs out at around six months. A baby's brain triples in size in the first year and a deficiency in iron can have a profound effect on learning later in life.

Pasta

Pasta tends to be a favorite with babies and young children. It's a good source of carbohydrates, and adding tiny pasta shapes to purées when your baby is about eight months is a good way to encourage chewing. Many vegetable purées make good pasta sauces, to which you could add a little grated cheese. Buy tiny pasta shapes like stars or shells. Also try quick-cook couscous, which has a soft texture perfect for babies. It is ready quickly and combines well with diced chicken or vegetables.

Textures

Problems with lumps are very common. Babies who are fed exclusively on jars often have a really difficult time progressing from smooth stage 1 foods to stage 2 jars, which often contain quite large lumps like whole peas.

This is too sudden a transition for them. It is important to introduce texture and small lumps as early as possible, as, the older they are, the harder babies will find it to accept lumpy food. This makes the transition to eating normal family meals a very difficult one and can lead to many toddler eating problems and extreme fussiness. One benefit (among many others) of making your own food is that this allows you to introduce lumps very gradually.

Another benefit of introducing lumpy food is that the muscles used to chew are the same muscles used for speech, so chewing will help with your baby's speech development. Even if your baby doesn't have many teeth, he can still chew using his gums.

Try thickening purées first of all, then adding lumps like really tiny pasta shapes, rice, or couscous. Also try mashing a portion of your baby's food, then adding it to the purée, gradually increasing the ratio of mashed to puréed food. Try finely chopping a few of the vegetables so that his puréed meal contains tiny lumps, but keep these very soft for a while so his gums can squash them when he tries to chew. Well-cooked scrambled eggs are another good way of introducing texture. Offering finger foods at this age is a good idea as many babies learn to eat lumps this way rather than in purées and this is fine.

Toast sticks, lightly steamed vegetable sticks, banana, tiny pieces of cheese (and later, sticks of cheese), grated apple, rice cakes, etc. are good finger foods.

The problem with organic jar baby foods is that they contain fewer natural vitamins and minerals than fresh foods. Studies have shown that babies fed on only organic baby food are at a higher risk of iron deficiency as no added iron is allowed in organic baby food. An infant fed exclusively on organic baby food would consume 20 percent less iron than one eating non-organic baby food.

Feeding pre-term babies

Babies born before 37 weeks are considered pre-term and have a greater need for certain nutrients like iron and zinc, because these only start to be stored in your baby's body in the last weeks of pregnancy. Pre-term babies tend to be in a state of catch-up so make sure you give lots of nutrient-dense foods like cheese, avocado, and potato.

Fruit

Going Bananas ☺ ☹

Babies love bananas and this recipe makes them taste truly scrumptious. It is delicious with vanilla ice cream. Try to use bananas with brown spots on the skin, as this shows they are ripe.

MAKES 1 PORTION
1 teaspoon butter
1 small banana, peeled and sliced
a pinch of ground cinnamon
2 tablespoons freshly squeezed orange juice

Melt the butter in a small skillet, stir in the sliced banana, sprinkle with a little cinnamon, and sauté for 2 minutes. Pour in the orange juice and continue to cook for another 2 minutes. Mash with a fork.

Banana and Blueberry ☺ ☹

Bananas combine well with lots of different fruits. Try also peach, mango, dried apricot, or prune. You can also mix banana and fruit combinations with some full-fat natural yogurt. Serve straight away, before the banana turns brown.

MAKES 1 PORTION
¼ cup blueberries
1 tablespoon water
1 small ripe banana, peeled and sliced

Put the blueberries into a saucepan with the water and cook for about 2 minutes or until the fruit just starts to burst open. Whiz with a hand (immersion) blender, together with the sliced banana, until smooth.

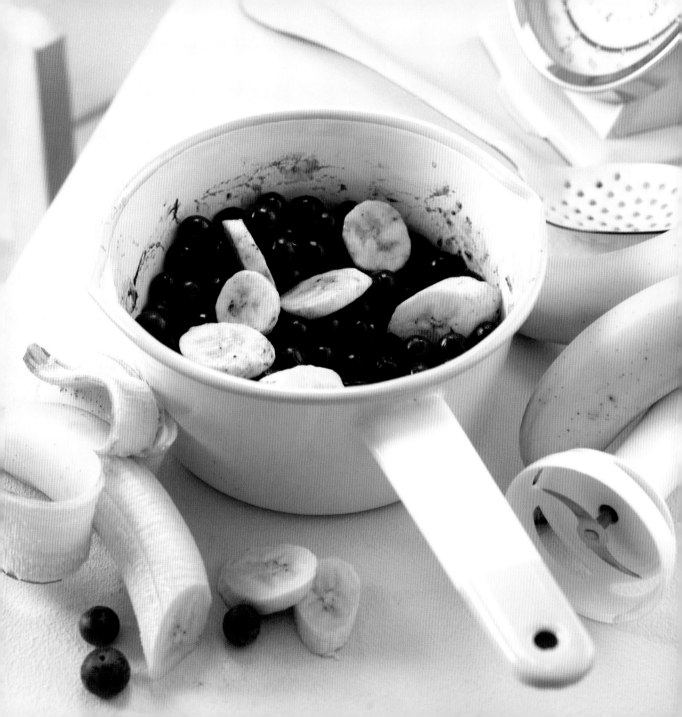

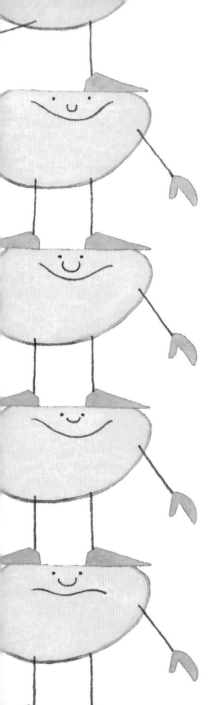

Peach, Apple, and Strawberry Purée ❄ ☺ ☹

You could also make Apple, Strawberry, and Blueberry Purée using ¼ cup blueberries instead of peach.

MAKES 2 PORTIONS
1 large apple, peeled, cored, and chopped
1 large ripe peach, peeled, pitted, and chopped
³⁄₄ cup strawberries, halved
1 tablespoon baby rice

Steam the apple for about 4 minutes. Add the peach and strawberries to the steamer and continue to cook for about 3 minutes. Blend the fruits to a smooth purée and stir in the baby rice.

Apple, Apricot, and Tofu ☺ ☹

Tofu is soya bean curd made from soya milk. It's a really good source of protein if you want to bring your child up on a vegetarian diet. It's also an excellent source of calcium, so adding tofu to fruit or vegetable purées is a good way to boost the calcium intake of babies who are allergic to cow's milk.

MAKES 2 PORTIONS
2 dessert apples, peeled, cored, and chopped
6 dried apricots, chopped
3 oz soft (silken) tofu

Place the apples and apricots in a pan and cover with water. Bring to the boil, reduce the heat, cover and simmer for about 5 minutes. Purée the fruit in a hand blender, together with the tofu.

Apricot, Apple, and Peach Purée ❄ ☺ ☹

Dried apricots are a concentrated source of nutrients, they are rich in iron, potassium and betacarotene, and babies tend to like their sweet flavor.

MAKES 5 PORTIONS

²/₃ cup ready-to-eat dried apricots (not Californian apricots)
2 dessert apples, peeled, cored, and chopped
1 large ripe peach, skinned, pitted, and chopped,
*   or 1 ripe pear, peeled, cored, and chopped*

Put the apricots into a small saucepan and cover with water. Cook over a low heat for 5 minutes. Add the chopped apples and continue to cook for 5 minutes. Purée together with the peach or pear.

Yogurt and Fruit ☺ ☹

It's important to make sure that, as well as fruit and vegetables, your baby gets enough fat in his diet. Recipes like vegetables in cheese sauce and fruit mixes with yogurt are very good for babies.

MAKES 1 PORTION

fresh fruit, e.g. 1 ripe peach, small mango, or a combination
*   like mango and banana*
2 tablespoons whole-milk natural yogurt
a little maple syrup (optional)

Peel the fruit, remove any pits, mash the flesh, and mix with the yogurt. Stir in a little maple syrup to sweeten if necessary.

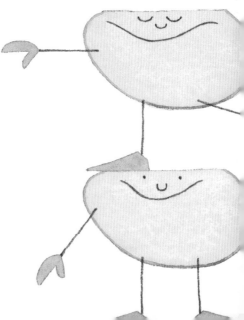

Vegetables

Lovely Lentils ❄ ☺ ☹

Lentils are a good cheap source of protein. They also provide iron, which is very important for brain development, particularly between the ages of six months and two years. Lentils can be difficult for young babies to digest and should be combined with plenty of fresh vegetables as in this recipe. This tasty purée also makes a delicious soup for the family by simply adding more broth and some seasoning.

MAKES 8 PORTIONS

½ small onion, finely chopped
1 cup carrot (4 oz), chopped
½ stalk celery (½ oz), chopped
1 tablespoon vegetable oil
¼ cup split red lentils
1¾ cups sweet potato, peeled and chopped
1¾ cups chicken or vegetable broth (see page 76 or 38) or water

Sauté the onion, carrot, and celery in the vegetable oil for about 5 minutes or until softened. Add the lentils and sweet potato and pour over the broth or water. Bring to a boil, turn down the heat, and simmer, covered, for 20 minutes. Purée in a blender.

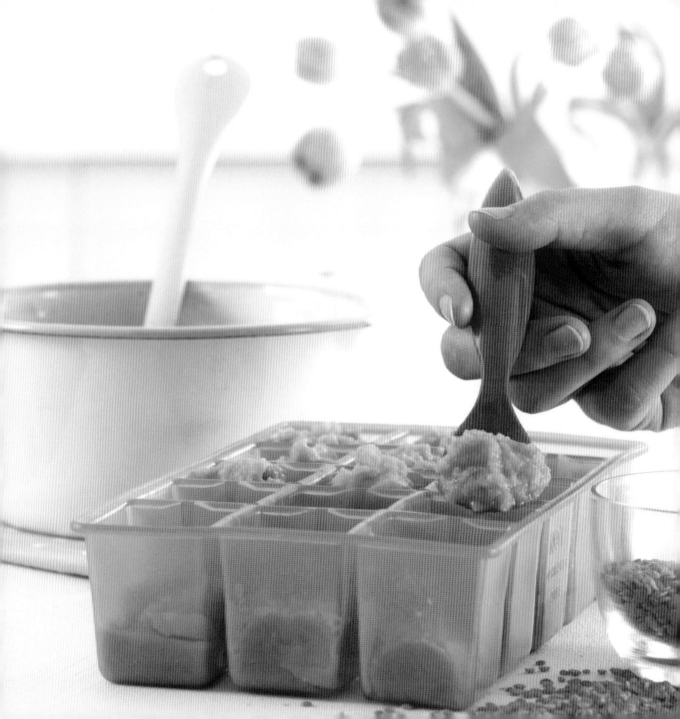

Tomatoes and Carrots with Basil ❄ ☺ ☹

If you introduce your baby to new flavors at an early age, he will tend to grow up a less fussy eater.

MAKES 4 PORTIONS
heaping 1 cup carrots, peeled and sliced
1 cup cauliflower florets
2 tablespoons butter
½ lb ripe tomatoes, skinned, seeded, and roughly chopped
2–3 fresh basil leaves
½ cup Cheddar cheese, grated

Put the carrots in a small saucepan, cover with boiling water, and simmer, covered, for 10 minutes. Add the cauliflower and cook, covered, for 7–8 minutes, adding extra water if necessary. Meanwhile, melt the butter, add the tomatoes, and sauté until mushy. Stir in the basil and cheese until melted. Purée the carrots and cauliflower with about 3 tablespoons of the cooking liquid and the tomato sauce.

Baked Sweet Potato with Orange ❄ ☺ ☹

Sweet potatoes are delicious baked like jacket potatoes either in the oven or microwave and then combined with fruit like apple or peach purée. They are a good source of carbohydrate, vitamins, and minerals.

MAKES 8 PORTIONS
1 medium sweet potato, scrubbed
2 tablespoons freshly squeezed orange juice
2 tablespoons milk

Cook the sweet potato on a cookie sheet in an oven preheated to 400°F for about 1 hour or until tender. Cool a little, then scoop out the flesh. Purée or mash with the orange juice and milk until smooth.

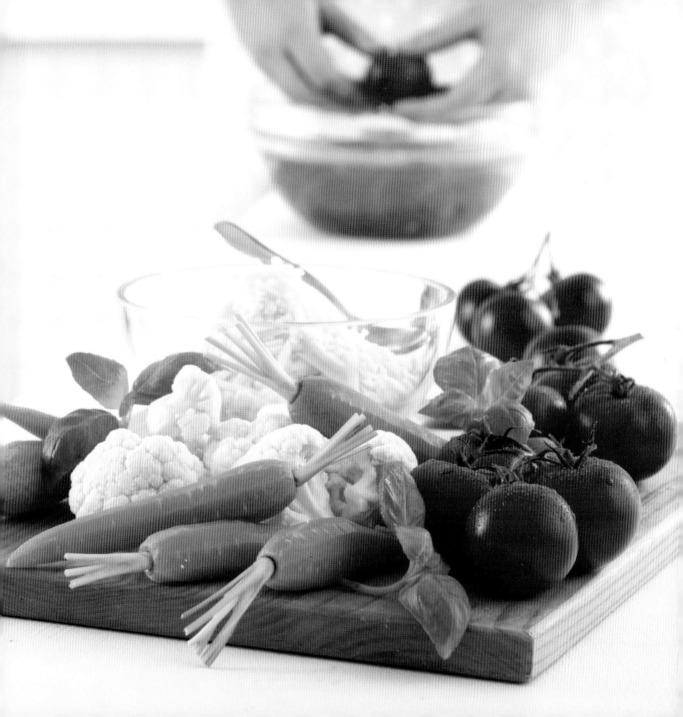

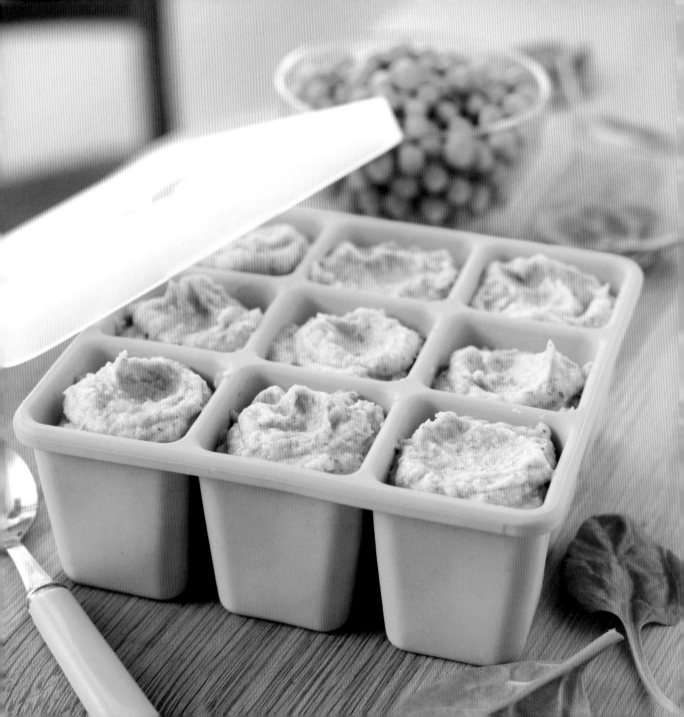

Sweet Potato, Spinach, and Peas ❄ ☺ ☹

This purée makes a tasty introduction to spinach for your baby.

MAKES 4 PORTIONS
2 teaspoons vegetable oil
a pat of butter
3 tablespoons finely chopped leek (white part only)
1 small garlic clove, crushed
1 cup peeled and diced sweet potato
1 cup peeled and diced potato
scant 1 cup boiling water
1¼ cups (loosely packed) fresh spinach
⅓ cup frozen peas
½ cup grated sharp Cheddar cheese

Heat the oil and butter in a saucepan and sauté the leeks for about 4 minutes, until softened. Add the garlic and sauté for 30 seconds. Add the sweet potato and potato and pour in the boiling water. Cook, covered, for 9 minutes. Add the spinach and peas and cook for 3 minutes. Remove from the heat and stir in the cheese until melted. Purée in a blender. If necessary, you can thin the purée with a little milk.

Sweet Vegetable Purée ❄ ☺ ☹

Peas and corn should be puréed in a food mill as the husks are indigestible.

MAKES 3 PORTIONS
2 tablespoons onion, chopped
³/₄ cup carrot, peeled and chopped
1 tablespoon olive oil
1¹/₄ cups potato, peeled and chopped
³/₄ cup plus 1 tablespoon water
2 tablespoons frozen corn
1 tablespoon frozen peas

Fry the onion and carrot gently in the oil for 5 minutes. Stir in the potato, add the water, bring to a boil, then cover and simmer for 10 minutes. Add the corn and peas and simmer for about 5 minutes. Purée in a food mill.

Trio of Cauliflower, Red Pepper, and Corn ❄ ☺ ☹

Babies like the bright color and natural sweetness of these vegetables. Always purée corn in a food mill for young babies, to get rid of the tough outer skin.

MAKES 4 PORTIONS
1 cup cauliflower florets
¹/₂ cup milk
¹/₂ cup Cheddar cheese, grated
¹/₄ small red bell pepper, chopped
¹/₂ cup frozen corn

Put the cauliflower in a small saucepan with the milk and cook over a low heat for about 8 minutes until tender. Stir in the grated cheese until melted. Meanwhile, steam the red pepper and corn or cook in some water in a small saucepan for about 6 minutes until tender. Strain the corn and pepper. Purée together with the cauliflower, milk, and cheese in a food mill.

Cauliflower Cheese ❄ ☺ ☹

This is a great favorite with babies. Try using different cheeses or combinations of cheese until you find your baby's preferred taste. The cheese sauce can be used over a mixture of vegetables as well.

MAKES 5 PORTIONS
1¹/₂ cups cauliflower florets

CHEESE SAUCE
1 tablespoon butter
1 tablespoon all-purpose flour
²/₃ cup milk
¹/₂ cup Cheddar, Edam, or Gruyère cheese, grated

Wash the cauliflower carefully and steam until tender (about 10 minutes). Meanwhile, for the sauce, melt the butter over a low heat in a heavy-bottomed saucepan and stir in the flour to make a smooth paste. Whisk in the milk and cook, stirring, until thickened. Take the saucepan off the heat and stir in the grated cheese. Keep stirring until all the cheese has melted and the sauce is smooth.

Add the cauliflower to the sauce and purée in a blender for younger babies. For older babies, mash with a fork or chop into little pieces.

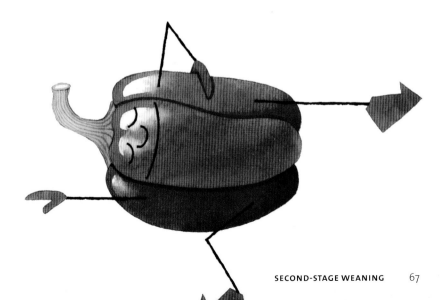

Zucchini Gratin ❄ ☺ ☹

This creamy purée is also good using broccoli.

MAKES 6 PORTIONS
1 medium potato (about ¹/₄ lb), peeled and chopped
1¹/₂ cups zucchini, sliced
a pat of butter
scant ¹/₂ cup Cheddar or Gruyère cheese, grated
¹/₄ cup milk

Boil the potato until soft. Steam the zucchini for 6–7 minutes. Strain the potatoes, add the butter and cheese, and stir until melted. Purée the potato mixture, zucchini, and milk with a hand (immersion) blender or mash for older babies.

Leek and Potato Purée ❄ ☺ ☹

This was Lara's favorite vegetable purée. It also makes a delicious soup for adults if you add seasoning.

MAKES 4 PORTIONS
2 tablespoons butter
heaping 1¹/₂ cups leeks, finely sliced
2¹/₄ cups potato, peeled and chopped
1¹/₄ cups chicken or vegetable broth (see page 76 or 38)
2 tablespoons Greek whole-milk yogurt

Heat the butter in a saucepan. Add the leeks and cook over a low heat for 5 minutes, stirring occasionally. Add the potatoes and pour over the broth. Cover and cook for about 12 minutes or until tender. Strain the vegetables and purée in a food mill or blender, adding as much of the cooking liquid as necessary to make a smooth consistency. Stir in the yogurt.

Carrot, Apple, and Spinach Purée ❄ ☺ ☹

A good way to introduce new vegetables is to mix them with familiar ones.

MAKES 3–4 PORTIONS
1 tablespoon olive oil
1½ cups grated carrot
1½ cups peeled, cored, and grated apple
2 cups (packed) baby spinach leaves, large stems removed

Heat the oil in a large saucepan and sauté the carrot for 5–6 minutes until starting to soften. Add the apple and ¼ cup water and bring to a boil. Reduce the heat and simmer for 8–10 minutes, until the carrot and apple are soft and the water has evaporated. Add the spinach leaves and 2 tablespoons more water and cook, stirring, until the spinach has wilted and the water has evaporated again. Cool and purée. If a slightly looser texture is required, you can purée the mixture with 2–3 tablespoons of your baby's usual milk.

Minestrone ❄ ☺ ☹

The vegetables in minestrone soup add texture but are nice and soft for your baby to chew. However, for younger babies you could blend this soup to the desired texture. Add a little seasoning and some extra broth to make this into a delicious soup for the rest of the family.

MAKES 4 ADULT PORTIONS OR 12 BABY PORTIONS
1 tablespoon vegetable oil
½ small onion, finely chopped
½ leek, white part only, washed and finely chopped
1 medium carrot, peeled and diced
½ celery stalk, diced
1 cup green beans, cut into ½-inch lengths
1 potato, peeled and diced
1 tablespoon fresh parsley, finely chopped
2 teaspoons tomato paste
1¼ quarts chicken or vegetable broth (see page 76 or 38)
3 tablespoons frozen peas
⅓ cup very small pasta shapes

Heat the oil in a saucepan and fry the onion and leek for 2 minutes, then add the carrot, celery, green beans, potato, and parsley and sauté for 4 minutes. Stir in the tomato paste and cook for 1 minute. Pour over the chicken or vegetable broth and simmer, covered, for 20 minutes. Add the frozen peas and pasta and cook for 5 minutes (check the box instructions for the cooking time of pasta).

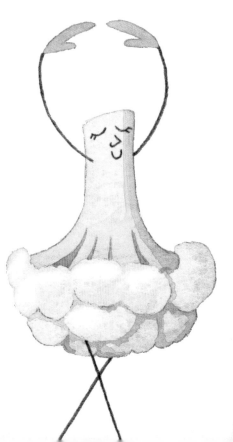

Fish

Tasty Fish with Cheese Sauce and Vegetables ❄ ☺ ☹

Fish and cheese sauce go really well together and the combination is always popular.

MAKES 6 PORTIONS
1 tablespoon butter
3/4 cup leek, thoroughly washed and finely sliced
1 medium carrot, peeled and chopped
heaping 1/2 cup broccoli florets
3 tablespoons frozen peas
5 oz cod fillets, skinned
2/3 cup milk
3 peppercorns
1 bay leaf

CHEESE SAUCE
1 1/2 tablespoons butter
1 tablespoon all-purpose flour
scant 1/2 cup Cheddar cheese, grated

Melt the butter in a saucepan, add the leeks, and sauté for 3 minutes. Add the carrot, cover with boiling water, and cook for 12 minutes. Add the broccoli and cook for 5 minutes. Stir in the peas and simmer for 3–4 minutes or until the vegetables are tender.

Meanwhile, put the fish in a pan with the milk, peppercorns, and bay leaf. Simmer for 4 minutes or until the fish is cooked. Strain, reserving the cooking liquid. Discard the peppercorns and bay leaf.

To prepare the sauce, melt the butter in a pan, stir in the flour, and cook for 1 minute. Gradually whisk in the milk in which the fish was cooked. Bring to a boil and cook, stirring until the sauce has thickened. Remove from the heat, add the cheese, and stir until melted.

Strain the vegetables and mix with the flaked fish and cheese sauce. Provided the vegetables are tender, this can be mashed or chopped for older babies who are starting to chew. Blend to a purée of the desired consistency for young babies.

Salmon with Carrots and Tomato ❄ ☺ ☹

This makes a good, creamy-textured fish purée.

MAKES 4 PORTIONS
2¼ cups carrot (½ lb), peeled and sliced
5 oz salmon fillet
½ tablespoon milk (or enough to cover the salmon, see method below)
2 tablespoons butter
2 medium, ripe tomatoes, skinned, seeded, and chopped
scant ½ cup Cheddar cheese, grated

Put the carrots in a steamer set over a pan of boiling water and cook for 15–20 minutes or until tender. Meanwhile, place the fish in a microwave dish, add the milk, dot with half the butter, and cover, leaving an air vent. Microwave on High for 1½–2 minutes until cooked. Alternatively, put the salmon in a pan, pour over enough milk to just cover, and simmer for about 4 minutes or until cooked.

Melt the remaining butter in a saucepan, add the tomatoes, and sauté until softened and slightly mushy. Remove from the heat and stir in the cheese until melted. Blend the cooked carrots with the tomato mixture. Drain the cooking liquor from the fish, remove the skin, and check there are no bones. Flake the fish and mix it with the carrots and tomatoes. For younger babies you can blend the fish together with the carrots and tomato for a smoother texture.

Oily fish like salmon provide the best source of essential fatty acids, which are very important for brain development – a baby's brain triples in size in the first year. A diet rich in EFAs can help children who have dyslexia, ADHD and dyspraxia. A lot of foods are now enriched with omega-3; however, most of these are plant-derived rather than fish oil-derived and are in quantities that provide little benefit. It is much better to concentrate on natural sources.

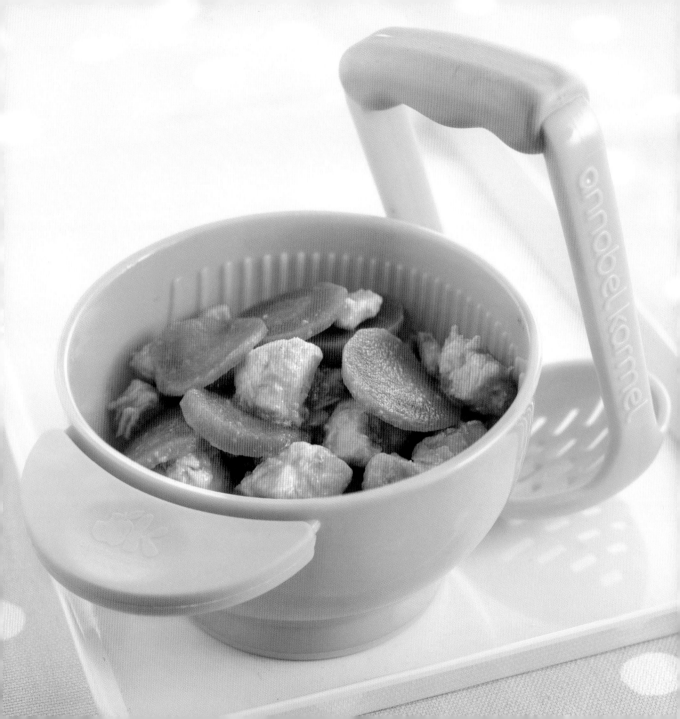

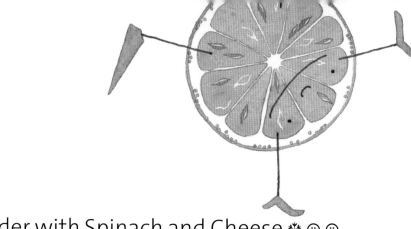

Flounder with Spinach and Cheese ❄ ☺ ☹

Frozen vegetables are a good alternative to fresh, and can often be more nutritious than vegetables that have been in the kitchen for several days. It also means you can make this when fresh spinach is not available.

MAKES 8 PORTIONS

½ lb flounder or grey sole fillets, skinned
1 tablespoon milk
1 bay leaf
a few peppercorns
a pat of butter
7 cups (6 oz) fresh or 1 cup frozen spinach

CHEESE SAUCE

2 tablespoons butter
2 tablespoons all-purpose flour
3/4 cup milk
½ cup Gruyère cheese, grated

Put the flounder in a suitable dish with the milk, bay leaf, peppercorns, and butter and microwave for about 3 minutes on High. Or, poach in a saucepan for 5 minutes. Meanwhile, cook the spinach in a saucepan with just a little water clinging to the leaves for about 3 minutes or cook frozen spinach following the box instructions. Squeeze out the excess water. Make the cheese sauce (see page 67). Discard the bay leaf and peppercorns, flake the fish carefully, and purée with the spinach and cheese sauce to the desired consistency.

Fillet of Cod with Sweet Potato ❄ ☺ ☹

The orange-fleshed sweet potato is an excellent source of beta carotene, which may help to prevent certain types of cancer.

MAKES 8 PORTIONS
2 cups sweet potato, peeled and diced
3 oz cod, skinned and filleted
2 tablespoons milk
a pat of butter
juice of 1 orange (about ½ cup)

Put the sweet potato into a saucepan, just cover with water, bring to a boil, then cover and simmer for 20 minutes or until soft. Put the fish in a suitable dish, add the milk, dot with butter, cover, and microwave on High for 2 minutes or until the fish is cooked. Alternatively, poach the fish in a saucepan with the milk and butter for 6–7 minutes or until just cooked through. Put the cooked sweet potato, strained fish, and orange juice into a blender and purée until smooth.

Fillet of Fish in an Orange Sauce ☺ ☹

Over the last 15 years this has been a very popular recipe – it has a lovely rich taste.

MAKES 5 PORTIONS
½ lb white fish fillets, skinned, e.g. cod or halibut
juice of 1 orange (about ½ cup)
scant ½ cup Cheddar cheese, grated
2 teaspoons fresh parsley, finely chopped
1 cup cornflakes, crushed
pat of butter or margarine, plus extra for greasing

Put the fish in a greased ovenproof dish, cover with the orange juice, cheese, parsley, and cornflakes and dot with the butter or margarine. Cover with aluminum foil and bake in an oven preheated to 350°F for about 20 minutes. Alternatively, cover with a lid and cook in a microwave on High for 4 minutes.

Flake the fish carefully, removing any bones, and mash everything together with the liquid in which the fish was cooked.

Chicken

Chicken Broth and My First Chicken Purée ❄ ☺ ☹

Bouillon cubes are unsuitable for babies under a year as they are high in salt, so I make my own chicken broth and use it as a base for chicken and vegetable purées. It keeps in the fridge for 3 days. For babies over one year you can add 3 chicken bouillon cubes for a stronger flavor, and you could also serve this as a soup with some noodles. Instead of an uncooked chicken, you could use the carcass from a roast chicken.

MAKES ABOUT 2½ QUARTS
1 large chicken, plus giblets
2¼ quarts water
2 parsnips
3 large carrots
2 leeks
2 large onions
1 celery stalk
2 sprigs of fresh parsley
1 bouquet garni

Cut the chicken into eight pieces, trimming off the excess fat. Trim, peel, wash, and chop the vegetables as necessary. Put the chicken pieces into a large saucepan together with the giblets. Cover with the water, bring to a boil and skim the froth from the top. Add the remaining ingredients and simmer for about 3 hours. It is best to remove the chicken breasts after about 1½ hours if you are going to eat them; otherwise they will become too dry.

Leave the broth in the refrigerator overnight and remove any congealed fat from the top in the morning. Strain out all the chicken and vegetables to complete the chicken broth.

You can purée some of the chicken breast in a food mill, together with a selection of the vegetables and some broth to make a chicken and vegetable purée. This also makes a wonderful clear chicken soup (with added bouillon cubes and seasoning) for older babies.

Chicken with Cottage Cheese ☺ ☹

Babies of this age are a little too young to eat pieces of chicken as finger food. This and the following three recipes show you simple ways of transforming cold chicken into tasty food for your baby.

MAKES 2 PORTIONS
¼ cup cooked boneless chicken (2 oz), chopped
1 tablespoon natural yogurt
1½ tablespoons cottage cheese with pineapple

Mix together the chicken, yogurt, and cottage cheese. Blend to the desired consistency.

Chicken Salad Purée ❄ ☺ ☹

What could be simpler? For toddlers, simply chop the ingredients, leave out the yogurt, and mix with mayonnaise.

MAKES 1 PORTION
2 tablespoons cooked boneless chicken (1 oz), chopped
1 slice cucumber, peeled and chopped
1 small tomato, skinned, seeded, and chopped
¼ cup avocado, peeled and chopped
1 tablespoon mild natural yogurt

Put all the ingredients into a blender and purée to the desired consistency. Serve immediately.

Chicken with Sweet Potato and Apple ❄ ☺ ☹

This combination gives a smooth texture and sweet taste that babies like.

MAKES 4 PORTIONS

1½ tablespoons vegetable oil
⅓ cup chopped onion
1 cup chopped chicken breast (about 4 oz)
½ apple, peeled and chopped
1 sweet potato (about 11 oz), peeled and chopped
1 cup chicken broth (see page 76)

Heat the oil in a saucepan, add the onion, and sauté for 2–3 minutes. Add the chicken and sauté until it turns opaque. Add the apple, sweet potato, and broth. Bring to a boil, cover, and simmer for 15 minutes. Purée to the desired consistency.

My First Chicken Stew with Peas ❄ ☺ ☹

This is an ideal purée for introducing young babies to chicken.

MAKES 4 PORTIONS

3 tablespoons finely chopped leek (white part only)
1 tablespoon butter
1 teaspoon vegetable oil
1 skinless, boneless chicken breast (about 6 oz), diced
heaping ½ cup peeled and diced carrot
1⅓ cups peeled and diced sweet potato
leaves from 2 sprigs fresh thyme
1 cup chicken broth (see page 76)
⅓ cup frozen peas

Sauté the leek in the butter and oil until softened. Add the chicken, carrot, sweet potato, and thyme and pour in the broth. Bring to a boil, then cover and simmer for about 15 minutes. Add the peas and continue to cook for 4 minutes. Remove from the heat and cool slightly. Purée.

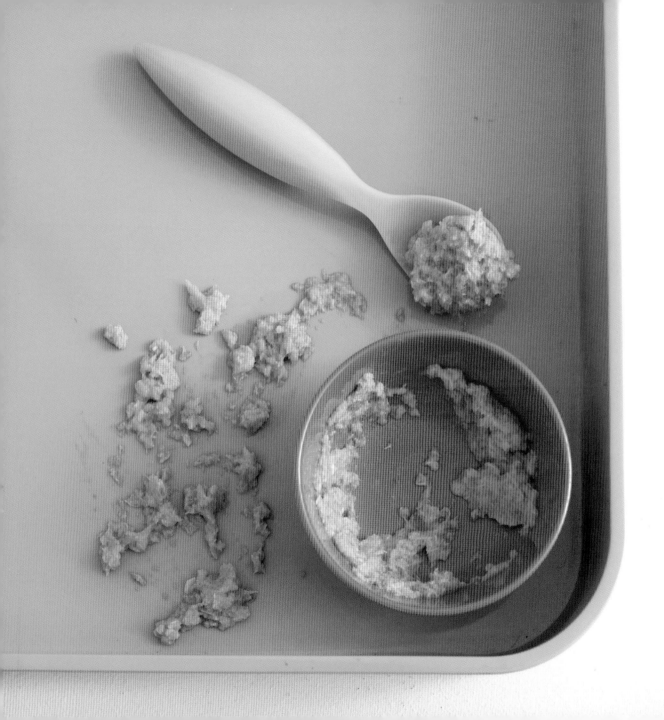

Chicken in Tomato Sauce ❄ ☺ ☹

MAKES 12 PORTIONS
¼ cup onion, chopped
1 cup carrot, thinly sliced
1½ tablespoons vegetable oil
1 small chicken breast (about ¼ lb), cut into chunks
1 cup potato, peeled and chopped
½ x 14-oz can diced tomatoes
⅔ cup chicken broth (see page 76)

Sauté the onion and carrot in the vegetable oil until softened, then add the chicken and potato and continue to cook for 3 minutes. Pour over the diced tomatoes together with the chicken broth. Bring to a boil and cook over a low heat for about 30 minutes or until the potato is quite soft. Put the mixture through a food mill or, for babies of nine months and older, chop in a blender. You could also add a little milk to make a smoother texture if you wish.

Fruity Chicken with Apricots ❄ ☺ ☹

Babies like the combination of chicken and fruit. Dried apricots are one of nature's great health foods. They are a good source of beta carotene, iron, and potassium, and the drying process increases their concentration. They also make great finger food. This is good by itself or you can mix it with ¼ cup of cooked rice or pasta.

MAKES 3 PORTIONS

2 teaspoons olive oil
½ small onion (⅓ cup), chopped
1 small garlic clove, crushed
chicken breast fillet, diced (⅓ cup)
1 cup peeled and diced sweet potato
3 dried apricots, chopped
⅔ cup tomato purée (no salt added)
⅔ cup chicken broth (see page 76) or water

Heat the oil in a pan and sauté the onion for about 5 minutes or until softened. Add the garlic and cook for 1 minute. Add the chicken and sauté for 2–3 minutes, until sealed. Add the sweet potato, apricots, tomato purée, and broth or water. Bring to a boil, then cover and simmer for about 5 minutes.

Red meats

Braised Beef with Sweet Potato ❄ ☺ ☹

Both this and the recipe below make good introductions to red meat.

MAKES 6 PORTIONS

1¼ tablespoons butter or margarine
1 leek, washed and sliced
¼ lb braising or stewing steak, cut into cubes
1 tablespoon flour
1¼ cups cremini mushrooms, sliced
2½ cups sweet potato, peeled and chopped
1 cup chicken broth (see page 76)
juice of 1 orange (about ½ cup)

Melt the butter or margarine in a Dutch oven and sauté the leek for about 4 minutes until softened. Roll the meat in the flour, add to the leek, and sauté until browned. Add the mushrooms and sauté for 1 minute. Add the sweet potato, broth, and orange juice. Bring to a boil and transfer to an oven, preheated to 350°F, for 1¼ hours, or until the meat is tender. Blend to the desired consistency using as much of the cooking liquid as necessary.

Liver Special ❄ ☺ ☹

MAKES 6 PORTIONS

3 oz calf's liver, or 2 chicken livers
½ cup chicken broth (see page 76)
½ cup leek, white part only, chopped
⅓ cup mushrooms, chopped
½ cup carrot, peeled and chopped
1 potato, peeled and chopped
a pat of butter
½ tablespoon milk

Trim and chop the liver and cook in the broth with the leek, mushrooms, and carrot for about 8 minutes over a low heat. Boil the potato until tender and mash with the butter and milk. Purée the liver and vegetables and mix with the potato.

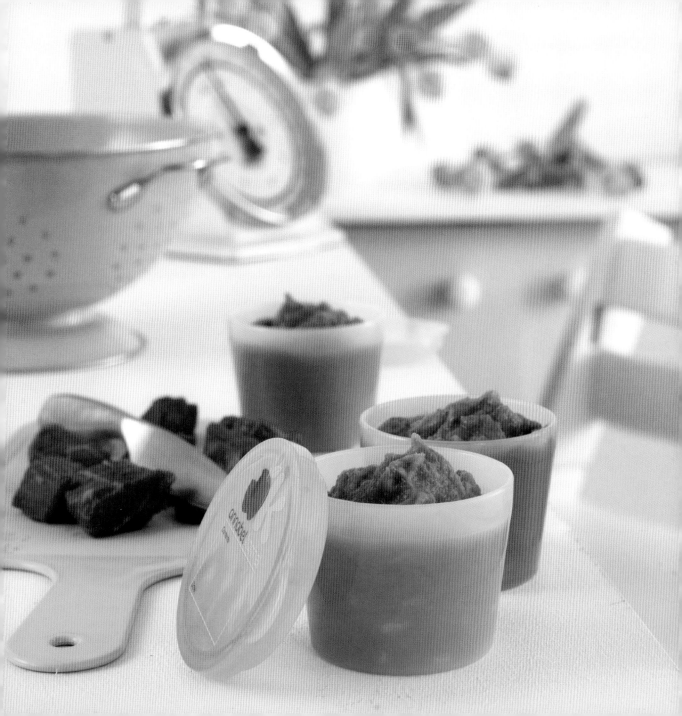

Pasta

Tomato and Butternut Squash Pasta Shells ❄ ☺ ☹

A tasty tomato sauce enriched with butternut squash and cheese.

MAKES 3 PORTIONS
³/4 cup peeled, coarsely chopped butternut squash
2 tablespoons small pasta shells
1 tablespoon butter
3 medium tomatoes, peeled, seeded, and cut into pieces
4 fresh basil leaves, torn into pieces
1 tablespoon crème fraîche or heavy cream

Steam the squash for 10 minutes, until tender. Meanwhile, cook the pasta following the package instructions. To make the tomato sauce, melt the butter and sauté the tomatoes for 3 minutes, until mushy. Stir in the basil. Blend the butternut squash with the tomato and basil. Stir in the crème fraîche or cream.

Vegetable and Cheese Pasta Sauce ❄ ☺ ☹

MAKES 3 PORTIONS OF SAUCE
³/4 cup carrot, peeled and sliced
heaping ¼ cup broccoli florets
2 tablespoons butter
2 tablespoons all-purpose flour
³/4 cup milk
scant ½ cup grated Cheddar cheese

Steam the carrot for 10 minutes, then add the broccoli florets and cook for 7 minutes more. Meanwhile, melt the butter in a small saucepan and stir in the flour to make a thick paste. Gradually add the milk, bring to a boil, and stir continuously until the sauce thickens. Simmer for 1 minute. Remove from the heat and stir in the grated cheese. Add the cooked vegetables to the cheese sauce and blend to a purée. Serve with tiny cooked pasta shapes.

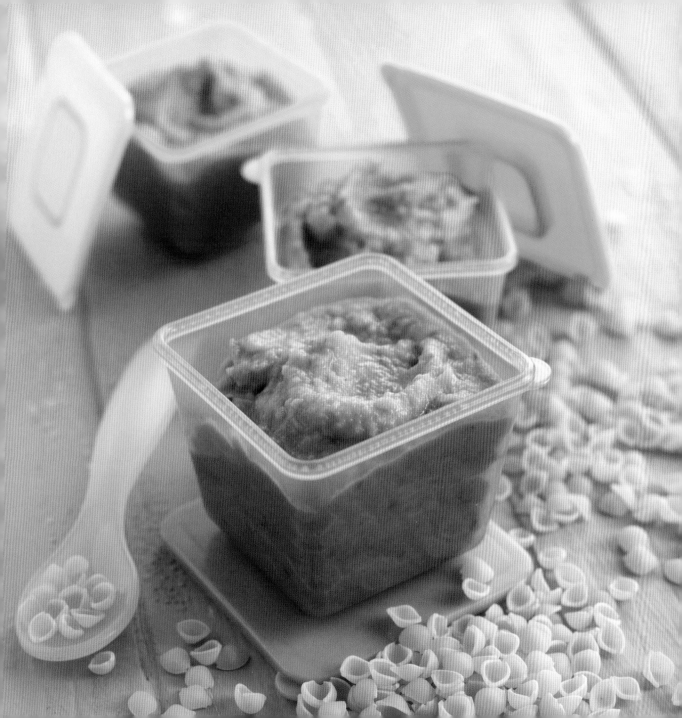

My First Bolognese Sauce ❄ ☺ ☹

MAKES 3 PORTIONS
1 tablespoon olive oil
1 small onion, peeled and chopped
1 garlic clove, crushed
1 medium carrot, peeled and grated
½ celery stalk, finely chopped
¼ lb lean ground beef
3 medium tomatoes, skinned and chopped
½ teaspoon tomato paste
⅔ cup unsalted chicken broth
3 tablespoons tiny pasta shapes

Heat the oil and sauté the onion, garlic, carrot, and celery for 5 minutes.
Add the ground beef and sauté until browned, stirring occasionally. Stir in
the tomatoes, tomato paste, and chicken broth. Bring to a boil, then simmer
for 15 minutes. Meanwhile, cook the pasta shapes following the box instructions.
Transfer the sauce to a blender and purée to a fairly smooth consistency. Drain
the pasta and mix with the sauce.

Tomato and Basil Pasta Sauce ❄ ☺ ☹

Butterfly-shaped pasta is fun for babies to grasp in their hands.

MAKES 2 PORTIONS
1 tablespoon butter
2 tablespoons onion, chopped
5 oz ripe tomatoes, skinned, seeded, and chopped
2 fresh basil leaves, torn
2 teaspoons cream cheese

Melt the butter in a saucepan and sauté the onion until softened. Add the
tomatoes and sauté for 3 minutes or until mushy. Stir in the basil and cream
cheese and heat through. Purée in a blender. Serve with cooked pasta of your
choice.

Napolitana Pasta Sauce ❄ ☺ ☹

A tasty tomato sauce which goes well with all types of pasta – my children love this with ravioli stuffed with ricotta and spinach.

MAKES 4 PORTIONS
1 tablespoon olive oil
½ small onion, peeled and chopped
½ garlic clove, peeled and crushed
½ cup carrot, peeled and diced
scant 1 cup tomato sauce with no added salt
3 tablespoons water
2 fresh basil leaves, roughly torn
1 teaspoon Parmesan cheese, grated
1 teaspoon cream cheese

Heat the olive oil and sauté the onion, garlic, and carrot for 6 minutes. Add the tomato sauce, water, basil, and Parmesan. Cover and simmer for 15 minutes. Purée the sauce and stir in the cream cheese. Mix with cooked pasta of your choice.

Popeye Pasta ❄ ☺ ☹

MAKES 4 PORTIONS
heaping 1 cup frozen or 9 cups fresh spinach, washed
(⅓ cup) tiny pasta stars or similar small pasta shapes
1 tablespoon butter
2 tablespoons milk
2 tablespoons cream cheese
scant ½ cup Gruyère cheese, grated

Cook the spinach following the box instructions or, if fresh, with just the water clinging to its leaves in a microwave or in a saucepan over a low heat until tender. Press out the excess water. Cook the pasta following the box instructions. Meanwhile, melt the butter in a small skillet and sauté the cooked spinach. Combine the spinach with the milk and cheeses, and chop finely in a food processor. Mix with the cooked pasta.

Second-stage weaning meal planner

	Breakfast	Mid-morning	Lunch	Mid-afternoon	Dinner	Bedtime
Day 1	Cheerios with milk Mashed banana Milk	Milk	**Chicken with Sweet Potato and Apple** Fruit* Juice	Milk	**Leek and Potato Purée** **Apricot, Apple, and Peach Purée** Water or juice	Milk
Day 2	Instant or homemade oatmeal with milk Fruit purée Milk	Milk	**Salmon with Carrots and Tomato** Mashed banana Juice	Milk	**Zucchini and Pea Soup** Yogurt Water or juice	Milk
Day 3	Apple purée and baby cereal Toast Milk	Milk	**Cauliflower Cheese** Fruit Juice	Milk	**Braised Beef with Sweet Potato** Baby crackers Water or juice	Milk
Day 4	Baby cereal with milk **Banana and Blueberry** Yogurt Milk	Milk	**Lovely Lentils** **Peaches and Rice** Juice	Milk	**Minestrone** Toast Water or juice	Milk

* Your baby should be able to hold and eat soft pieces of fruit

	Breakfast	Mid-morning	Lunch	Mid-afternoon	Dinner	Bedtime
Day 5	Cheerios with milk **Peach, Apple, and Strawberry Purée** Milk	Milk	Pasta with **Vegetable and Cheese Pasta Sauce** **Going Bananas** Juice	Milk	**My First Bolognese Sauce** Pear purée Water or juice	Milk
Day 6	Baby cereal with milk **Peach, Apple, and Strawberry Purée** Milk	Milk	**Tomatoes and Carrots with Basil** Fruit Juice	Milk	**Fillet of Fish in an Orange Sauce** Fruit Water	Milk
Day 7	Instant or homemade oatmeal with milk **Yogurt and Fruit** Milk	Milk	**Sweet Potato with Spinach and Peas** **Apricot, Apple, and Peach Purée** Juice	Milk	**My First Chicken Stew with Peas** **Apricot, Apple, and Peach Purée** Water or juice	Milk

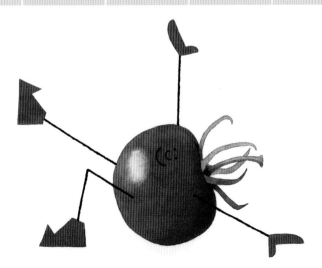

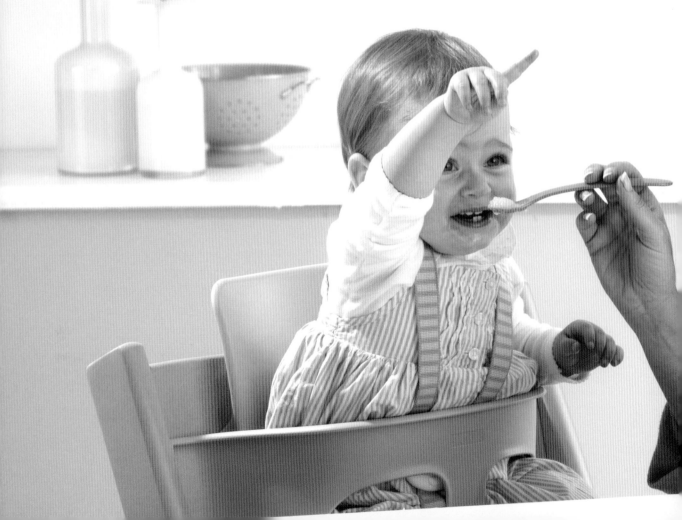

CHAPTER FOUR

Nine to twelve months

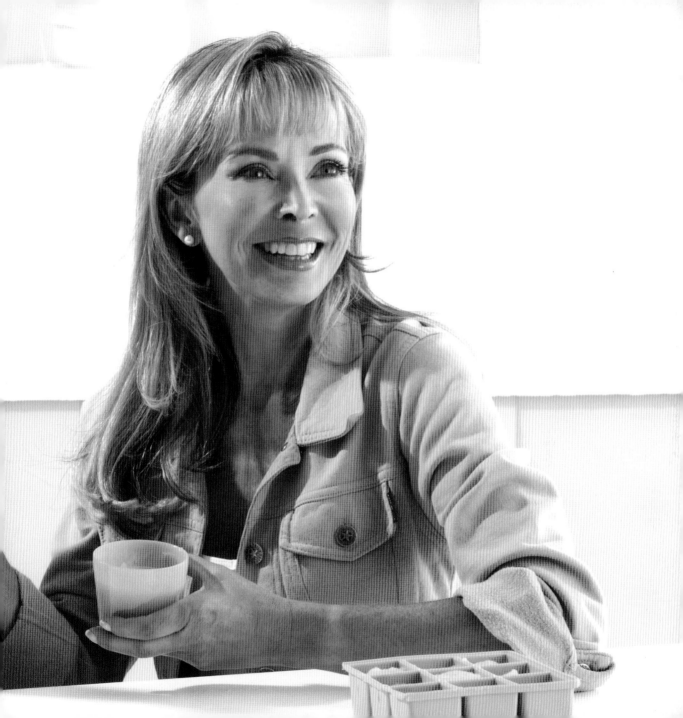

Towards the end of the first year, a baby's weight gain usually slows down quite dramatically. Often babies who have been good eaters in the past become much more difficult to feed. Try to give your baby her meals in a highchair at the table. Try to eat together, and make mealtimes fun and sociable. If she can see everyone around her eating happily, it is likely that she will want to join in.

This can be a difficult stage for many parents – babies find it hard to cope with more lumpy food and generally prefer to feed themselves than be fed, though their aim is often far from perfect! Interestingly, while many babies refuse anything with lumps in it, they will happily chew on finger foods like carrot or cucumber sticks, or pieces of fruit. Try nutritious finger foods like Chicken and Apple Balls (page 122), Salmon Footballs (page 120) or Fresh Fruit Ice Pops (page 108) – good for soothing sore gums.

Mealtime patience

Let your baby experiment by allowing her to use a spoon. Most of the food will probably end up on you or on the floor, but the more you allow your baby to experiment, the quicker she will master the art of feeding herself. Put a plastic splash mat under the highchair to catch the food that falls on the floor so that you can recycle it. It is probably best to have two bowls of food and two spoons; one which you use to spoon-feed your baby, the other (preferably a bowl which sticks to the table by suction) for your baby to play with. You will need lots of patience at

mealtimes, as many babies are very easily distracted at this stage and prefer to play with their food rather than eat it. If all else fails, I find that if you can attract their attention by giving them a small toy to hold, you can sometimes slip food into their mouths on a spoon, and they will eat without really noticing what they are doing and forget to put up any resistance!

Toddlers often go into "meltdown" just before dinner, especially if there has been some delay. Just before "meltdown" is a good time to offer some cut-up vegetables like carrots, cucumber, or peppers. If they haven't been snacking, they will be hungry and therefore more likely to eat them, and if they do get full, they will be full on vegetables, which is great. Just because a child doesn't like cooked vegetables doesn't mean they won't like the same vegetable raw, so always try both versions. Rather than chopping the vegetables and fruit into small pieces, I find that sometimes children prefer to be given a whole carrot or a chunk of cucumber.

Continue giving breast or infant formula milk as your baby's main drink. Cow's milk is not suitable as a main drink because it is low in essential vitamins and minerals like iron. However, as solid-food intake increases, milk need no longer form such a staple part of your child's diet, although they should still be drinking about 18 oz (2¼ cups) of milk a day (or the equivalent as dairy products or in cooking). It is an important source of protein and calcium. Many mothers assume that when their baby cries it is because she wants more milk, but often babies of this age are given too much milk and not enough solid food. If you fill your baby's stomach with milk when she really wants some solid food, you will not get a very satisfied baby.

Whilst it is a good idea to switch off the TV and try to provide a calm atmosphere, there is no doubt that there are some babies who will eat much better with the gentle distraction of a simple (washable) toy at the highchair. Some babies are much easier to feed if their hands are occupied, so giving your baby a spoon to hold is also worth a try …

If you have a juicer, you can make all sorts of wonderful fruit and vegetable drinks for your baby – try combinations like apple, strawberry, and banana. Your baby should now be drinking happily from a cup, the bottle kept for her bedtime drink of warm milk.

Your baby will be teething at this age and, very often, sore gums can put her off eating for a while. Don't worry, as she will make up for this later that day or the next day. (Rubbing a teething gel on your baby's gums, or giving her something very cold to chew, can help relieve soreness and restore appetite.)

It is a good idea to eat something with your baby at mealtimes. There are some mothers who sit opposite their babies and try to spoon food into their mouths whilst eating nothing themselves. Babies are great mimics and will be much more likely to enjoy eating if they see you tucking in as well.

When learning to feed themselves, babies should be allowed to smear food and generally make a mess.

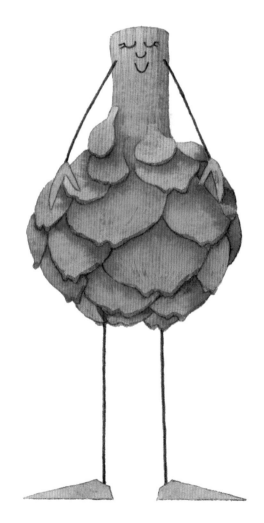

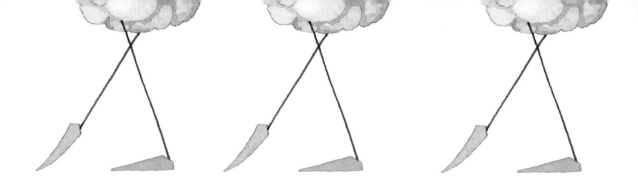

Make mealtimes a positive experience. Many babies hate having their faces wiped, so only wipe at the end of a meal unless they get themselves into a real mess. Try to wipe their face or hands with a flannel and warm water rather than baby wipes as the alcohol can sting any little sore areas on their chins from teething.

The foods to choose

Now you can be a little more adventurous with the food that you make for your baby. It is a good idea to develop her tastes for garlic and herbs, both of which are very healthy. Children tend to be less fussy eaters if they are introduced to a wide range of foods early. Again, if your baby dislikes certain foods, never force her to eat them; just leave out those foods and perhaps reintroduce them in a couple of days' time. Try also to vary the foods as much as possible, as this will lead to a more balanced diet. If you give your child a favorite food too often, it is possible she will go off it altogether.

Your baby can now eat berry fruits (these can be strained to get rid of the indigestible seeds). Fruit gelatins will be interesting for your baby to look at, feel, and eat. Your baby should also like fruit and vegetables that have been grated.

Oily fish like salmon, sardines, and fresh tuna should be included in your baby's diet as they contain essential fatty acids and iron that are important for the brain and visual development. Fish is quite simple to cook and if you use my recipes it is easy to make it appealing to your baby. All fish must obviously be very fresh.

When possible, try to make your baby's food look attractive on the plate. Choose colorful fruit and vegetables and make shapes like little faces. Don't pile too much food onto the plate and use mini-ramekin dishes to make individual portions of shepherd's pie or fish pie (you can also freeze them).

Meat

Red meat is good for young children as it provides the best source of iron. If using fresh ground meat, choose good-quality meat and ask your butcher to prepare it for you rather than buying it ready prepared. After cooking ground meat for young babies, I find that if I chop it in a food processor for 30 seconds, it becomes softer and easier to chew. At this age it is good to mix meat with tiny pasta shapes or rice. It is best not to give sausages or other processed meats like pâté or meat pies to children. The cocktail meatballs on page 180 would make excellent finger food.

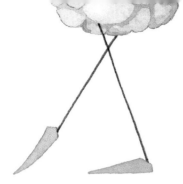

Textures and quantities

It is easy to get into the habit of only giving your baby soft foods, but you should try to vary the consistency of the food you offer. There is no need to purée all foods. Babies do not need teeth to be able to chew; gums do a great job on foods that are not too hard. Give some food mashed (fish), some grated (cheese), some diced (carrots) and some whole (pieces of chicken, slices of toast, and pieces of raw fruit).

As far as quantities are concerned, you must let your baby's appetite be your guide. You can start to freeze food in larger plastic containers and freeze individual portions like mini shepherd's pies in small ramekin dishes. Many meals in this chapter can be enjoyed by the whole family, in which case adult-sized portions are given.

Finger foods

By the age of nine months, your baby will probably want to start feeding herself. It is a good idea, therefore, to start giving her some foods that are easy to eat with her fingers. Finger foods are great for keeping your child occupied while you prepare her meal – or you could make a whole meal of finger foods.

Never leave your child unattended whilst eating. It is easy for a baby to choke on even very small pieces of food. Avoid giving your baby whole nuts, fruits that contain pits, whole grapes, ice cubes, olives, or any other foods that might get stuck in her throat.

What to do if your baby chokes

If your baby chokes, lay her face down on your forearm or lap with her head lower than her chest. Support her head and give her five light slaps between her shoulders with your free hand.

Fruit and ice pops

When giving your baby fruit, make sure it has been peeled and any pips or pits have been removed. If she finds it difficult to chew, give soft fruits that melt in the mouth such as bananas, peaches, or grated fruits. Berry and citrus fruits should only be given in small quantities to start with. Remove as much pith as possible.

Many babies who are teething really enjoy biting into something cold as this soothes sore gums. Try making fresh fruit ice pops: fill ice-pop molds with tasty combinations of puréed fruit, fruit juices, smoothies, and yogurt.

Dried fruits

These are a good source of fiber, iron, and energy. Choose ready-to-eat fruits that are soft and cut into very small pieces to reduce the risk of choking. Some dried apricots are treated with sulphur dioxide to preserve their bright orange color; these should be avoided as they can trigger an asthma attack in susceptible babies. Don't give your baby lots of dried fruit as it can be difficult to digest – and laxative.

Fruity ideas

Apple, apricot, avocado, banana, blueberries, cherries, clementine, grapes, kiwi fruit, mango, melon, nectarine, orange, papaya, peach, pear, plum, raspberries, strawberries, tomato

More fruity ideas

Chopped apple rings, dried apricots, banana chips, dates, dried pears, prunes, raisins, sultanas

Vegetables

To begin with, give your baby soft cooked vegetables cut into pieces that are easy for her to hold, and encourage her to bite off little pieces. (It is best to steam vegetables as this will help to preserve vitamin C.) Gradually cook the vegetables for less time so that your baby gets used to having to chew harder. Once your baby has good coordination, she will enjoy picking up little vegetables like peas and corn.

When your baby has mastered the art of feeding herself cooked vegetables, you can introduce raw vegetables. Even if your baby is unable to bite into these sticks, she will enjoy chewing on them as an aid to teething. In fact, sticks of raw vegetables such as carrots and cucumber are very soothing for sore gums if they are chilled in the freezer or in iced water for a few minutes. Large pieces of raw vegetables are safer than small pieces as a baby will nibble off what she can manage, whereas a small piece put into her mouth whole could cause her to choke if she tried to swallow it.

Once your baby can chew well, try giving her corn on the cob. Cut the corn in half or into three pieces. Corn is fun to eat and babies love to hold and chew it.

Vegetables are also very good when dipped into sauces and purées. Try using some of the recipes for vegetable purées as dipping sauces.

Keep a supply of puréed vegetables in the freezer, stored in ice-cube trays. Include favorites like butternut squash, sweet potato, and carrot and pea and some that your child may not be so keen on like zucchini, spinach, or broccoli. Defrost the amount you need and add them to popular dishes.
❀ Mix them with pasta sauce and tiny pasta shapes
❀ Hide in cheesy mashed potato
❀ Use as a spread in grilled cheese sandwiches.

Breads and teething biscuits

Pieces of toast, teething biscuits, and firm bread, like pitta bread and bagels, make good finger food and can be dipped into purées and sauces. Rice cakes come in lots of different flavors and are excellent for teething, as they seem to hold together well. You can also make broiled cheese on toast or spread toast with no-sugar conserves.

Many baby teething biscuits on the market contain as much sugar as a sweet cookie and even so-called low-sugar teething biscuits can contain more than 15 percent sugar. It is very easy to make your own sugar-free alternative from whole-grain bread (see below).

Vegetable finger food
Broccoli, carrots, cauliflower, celery, corn on the cob, zucchini, mushrooms, baby potatoes, sweet potato

Homemade teething biscuits
For homemade savory teething biscuits, simply cut a thick (½ inch) slice of whole-grain (granary or rye) bread into three strips. Melt ⅛ teaspoon Marmite or Vegemite in 1 teaspoon boiling water and brush evenly over the bread strips. Bake in an oven preheated to 350°F for 15 minutes. If your baby prefers, substitute a little grated cheese for the Marmite or Vegemite. You can prepare a store of teething biscuits in advance and keep them in an airtight container for 3–4 days.

Miniature sandwiches
Little sandwiches cut into fingers, squares, small triangles or even animal shapes using a cookie cutter are very popular with babies. Some suggestions for sandwich fillings are given below; use your imagination to come up with original, tasty combinations.

Filling suggestions
Mashed banana and/or peanut butter, tuna with canned corn and mayonnaise, hummus, cottage cheese with pineapple, cream cheese with strawberry preserve or chopped dried apricots, grated cheese and tomato, mashed sardines with tomato ketchup, egg mayonnaise and alfalfa sprouts

Breakfast cereals
Babies love to pick up and eat little pieces of breakfast cereal like Cheerios. Try to choose cereals that are fortified with iron and vitamins and which do not have added sugar. Again, some suggestions are given below.

Cheese
Start by giving your baby grated cheese or cut wafer-thin slices. Once she has mastered chewing, you can move on to chunks and strips of cheese. I have found that the following cheeses are especially popular: Cheddar, mozzarella, Edam, Gouda, Emmenthal, and Gruyère. Cream cheese and cottage cheeses are also favorites. Keep away from strong cheeses like blue cheese, Brie, and Camembert. Always make sure that the cheese you give your baby is pasteurized.

Good morning munchies
Cheerios, cornflakes, granola, Chex

Pasta

Pasta comes in all shapes and sizes, including tiny stars, mini shells, and animal and alphabet shapes. I have given some recipes for pasta sauces but most of the vegetable purées can also be served with pasta. You can try tossing pasta in melted butter and sprinkling with grated cheese. This is usually a great favourite, even with the fussy eaters.

Chicken

Slices or chunks of cooked chicken (or turkey) make great finger food. Give the dark meat as well as the white as it contains twice as much zinc and iron. Bang Bang Chicken and Chicken with Cornflakes (see page 124) are particularly good given as finger food.

Fish

Pieces of flaked white fish are good as they are low in fat, high in protein, and easy for your child to chew. You can give them to your baby either plain or mixed with a sauce. Make your own fish sticks by cutting white fish fillets into strips, coating in flour, beaten egg, and crushed cornflakes and then frying until golden. You could also try the Salmon Footballs on page 120. Do take extra care when serving fish to your baby in any recipe to check the fish thoroughly for bones before you cook it and when flaking it. Make sure you include some oily fish like salmon or sardines in your child's diet, preferably twice a week.

Breakfast

The first meal of the day is important for all of us after a night's fasting, particularly so for energetic babies and toddlers!

For this age group, recipes can now contain more interesting and more healthy grains. Wheatgerm is particularly good and can be sprinkled onto cereals or yogurt. Mixing cereals and fruit makes a delicious and nutritious start to the day. Many of the homemade cereals can be mixed with apple juice instead of milk.

Cheese is important for strong bones and teeth. You can offer broiled cheese on toast or little strips of cheese for your baby to hold. Eggs are an excellent source of protein, vitamins, and iron. Give your baby scrambled eggs or an omelet but make sure that the white and yolk are cooked until solid. Fresh fruit provides vitamins, minerals, and substances called phytochemicals which help prevent cancer. Give fruit as finger foods, make fruit salads, or offer stewed fruit, such as apple or rhubarb.

Highly refined, sugar-coated cereals should be avoided. Do not be fooled by the list of added vitamins on the side of the packet – unprocessed cereals are much healthier for your child. Whole-grain cereals are also a good source of iron, but you will need to include some vitamin C such as diluted orange juice or strawberries in order for your baby to absorb the iron.

Breakfast

Fruity Swiss Muesli ☺ ☹

This tasty and nutritious breakfast will make a good start to the day for the whole family. You can vary the fruit in the muesli, adding, for example, peaches, strawberries, bananas, or ready-to-eat dried apricots.

MAKES 4 CHILD OR 2 ADULT PORTIONS
$3/4$ cup quick-cook oats (not instant)
2 tablespoons wheatgerm
$2/3$ cup apple juice
1 teaspoon lemon juice
1 dessert apple, peeled and grated
1 pear, peeled, cored, and chopped
1 tablespoon maple syrup
$1/2$–$2/3$ cup natural yogurt

Combine the rolled oats, wheatgerm, and apple juice. Set aside for a couple of hours or refrigerate overnight. Next morning, mix the lemon juice with the grated apple and stir this into the oat mixture together with the chopped pear, maple syrup, and yogurt.

Fruity Yogurt ☺ ☹

Many commercial fruit yogurts have a lot of added sugar. It is easy to make your own, adding a combination of your baby's favorite foods.

MAKES 2 PORTIONS
$1/2$ ripe peach, pitted, skinned, and chopped
$1/2$ small banana, peeled and chopped
$2/3$ cup natural yogurt
2 teaspoons maple syrup

Simply mix all the ingredients together and serve. Mash the fruit for younger babies.

My Favorite Crêpes ❄ ☺ ☹

Crêpes for breakfast are a treat, and this simple recipe is foolproof. Crêpes can be made in advance, refrigerated, and reheated. To freeze, interleave with parchment paper. Serve with maple syrup and fresh fruit.

MAKES 12 CRÊPES
Heaping 3/4 cup all-purpose flour
generous pinch of salt (optional for babies over 1 year)
2 eggs
1 1/4 cups milk
3 tablespoons butter, melted

Whisk the flour and salt, if using, together in a mixing bowl, make a well in the center, and add the eggs. Use a balloon whisk to incorporate the eggs into the flour and gradually whisk in the milk until just smooth.

Brush a heavy-based 6–7-inch skillet with the melted butter and, when hot, pour in about 2 tablespoons of the batter. Quickly tilt the pan from side to side to form a thin layer of batter and cook for 1 minute. Flip the crêpe over with a spatula and cook until the underside is slightly golden. Continue with the rest of the batter, brushing the pan with melted butter when necessary.

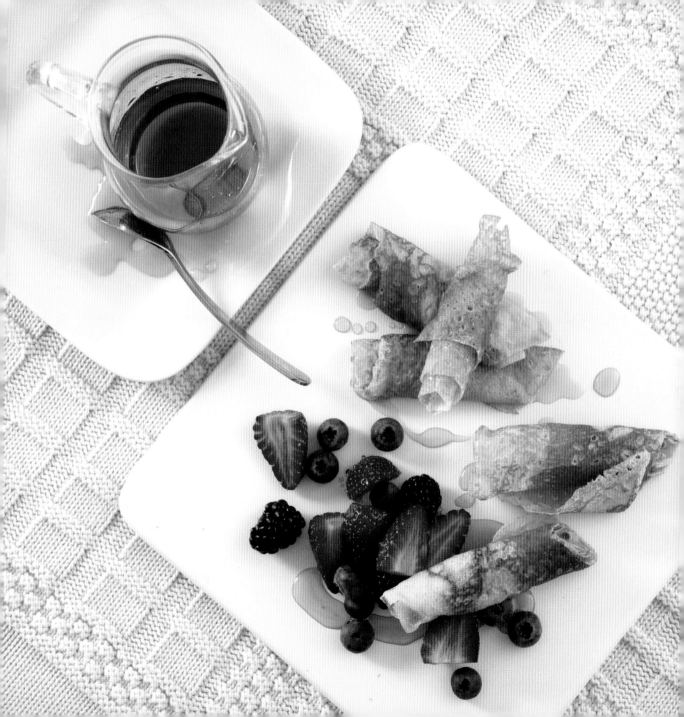

Apricot, Apple, and Pear Custard ❄ ☺ ☹

Dried apricots are one of nature's great health foods. They are a good concentrated source of beta carotene, potassium, and iron. This tasty fruit purée works well for breakfast or dessert.

MAKES 3 PORTIONS
½ cup ready-to-eat dried apricots, chopped
1 large dessert apple, peeled, cored, and chopped
1 tablespoon cornstarch
¼ teaspoon vanilla extract
⅔ cup milk
1 ripe pear, peeled, cored, and chopped

Gently heat the apricots and apple in a small saucepan with 4 tablespoons of water for 8–10 minutes or until soft. In a saucepan, blend the cornstarch and vanilla with a little of the milk to make a smooth paste. Then add the remaining milk and slowly bring to the boil, stirring until thickened and smooth. Blend the cooked fruit and pear to the desired consistency and stir in the custard.

A Grown-up Breakfast ☺ ☹

Unfortunately, many of the breakfast cereals designed specifically for children are laden with sugar. I prefer to give my children some of the more old-fashioned cereals like Weetabix, oatmeal, or muesli and sweeten these with fresh fruit.

MAKES 1 PORTION
½ Weetabix
1 small banana
3 tablespoons mild natural yogurt or milk

Finely crumble the Weetabix and mash the banana. Combine all the ingredients together and serve.

Summer Fruit Muesli ☺ ☹

Simply soak the oats overnight and stir in extra fresh fruits like peaches or strawberries the next day for a tasty nutritious muesli. If your baby is too young for lumpy food, this can be blended to a fine purée.

MAKES 4 ADULT PORTIONS
heaping 1 cup quick-cook oats
2 tablespoons raisins or golden raisins, chopped
1¼ cups apple and mango juice
2 dessert apples, peeled, cored, and grated
4–6 tablespoons milk
a little maple syrup (or honey, for babies over 1 year)

Mix the oats, raisins, and apple and mango juice in a bowl, cover, and leave to soak overnight in the refrigerator. In the morning, stir in the remaining ingredients and any extra fruit and drizzle over a little maple syrup or honey (if using).

Banana and Prune Fool ☺ ☹

This only takes a couple of minutes to prepare and it is very tasty. It is also a good recipe to try if your baby is a little bit constipated.

MAKES 1 PORTION
5 canned prunes in fruit juice, pitted
1 small ripe banana, peeled
1 tablespoon natural yogurt
1 tablespoon cream cheese

Whiz the prunes, banana, yogurt, and cream cheese together in a blender with 1–2 tablespoons of the juice from the canned fruit.

The Three Bears' Breakfast ☺ ☹

This makes a very nutritious breakfast, but make sure your child gobbles it up before Goldilocks comes to the front door!

MAKES 2 ADULT PORTIONS
1¼ cups milk
½ cup quick-cook oats (not instant)
2 tablespoons ready-to-eat dried peaches or apricots, chopped
1 teaspoon raisins, chopped

Pour the milk into a saucepan and bring to a boil. Mix in the oats and bring back to a boil, stirring. Add the chopped dried fruit, lower the heat, and simmer for about 4 minutes or until thickened.

Matzo Brei ☺ ☹

For those of you who have never heard of matzo, it is a large square of unleavened bread similar to crispbread. When uncooked, it is very brittle and my son Nicholas loved to snap it into pieces and strew it all over the floor. This is why I prefer to serve it cooked!

MAKES 2 ADULT PORTIONS
2 matzos
1 egg, beaten
2 tablespoons butter
a little sugar (optional)

Break the matzos into bite-sized pieces and soak for a couple of minutes in cold water. Squeeze out the excess water, then add the matzos to the beaten egg. Melt the butter in a skillet until sizzling and fry the matzos on both sides. Sprinkle with sugar if wished.

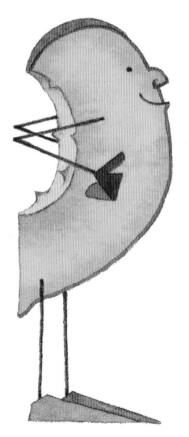

French Toast Cutouts ☺ ☹

It's sometimes fun to cut the bread into a variety of animal shapes using cookie cutters. For a treat, serve with maple syrup or fruit preserves.

MAKES 2 PORTIONS
1 egg
2 tablespoons milk
a pinch of ground cinnamon (optional)
2 slices white or raisin bread
2 tablespoons butter

Beat the egg lightly with the milk and cinnamon, if using, and pour into a shallow dish. Dip the bread in this mixture, coating each side. Melt the butter and fry the slices or animal shapes until golden on both sides.

Cheese Scramble ☺ ☹

Until your child is one year, scrambled egg should be cooked until it is quite firm and not runny. You could use cottage cheese instead of Cheddar.

MAKES 1 PORTION
1 egg
1 tablespoon milk
1 tablespoon butter
1 tablespoon Cheddar cheese, finely grated
1 tomato, skinned, seeded, and chopped

Beat the egg with the milk. Melt the butter in a saucepan over a low heat, then add the egg mixture. Cook slowly, stirring all the time. When the mixture has thickened and looks soft and creamily set, add the cheese and tomato. Serve immediately.

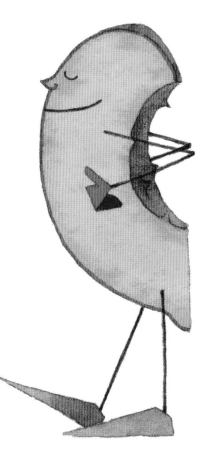

Fruit

Mini Banana Muffins ❄ ☺ ☹

These delicious mini muffins are perfect for breakfast or a snack at any time of the day, and are great for little hands.

MAKES 12 MINI MUFFINS
1 banana, as ripe as possible, mashed
2 tablespoons vegetable oil
1 egg yolk
½ teaspoon vanilla extract
3 tablespoons whole-wheat flour
3 tablespoons all-purpose flour
¼ teaspoon baking soda
¼ teaspoon ground cinnamon
pinch of salt (not for under ones)
2 tablespoons chopped raisins

Preheat the oven to 350°F. Line a mini muffin pan with 12 paper liners.

Whisk together the banana, oil, egg yolk, and vanilla. In a separate bowl, whisk together the flours, baking soda, cinnamon, salt (if using), and raisins. Add the banana mixture and stir until just combined.

Spoon into the prepared pan and bake for 10–12 minutes, until the muffins are risen and firm to the touch.

Cool for 5 minutes in the pan, then transfer to a wire rack and let cool completely.

Apple and Blackberry ❄ ☺ ☹

Blackberries and apples make a delicious combination, and the blackberries (which are rich in vitamin C) turn the apples a wonderful purple color. Instead of blackberries you could use other berry fruits like strawberries or blueberries, or a mixture.

MAKES 6 PORTIONS
2 tart apples, peeled, cored, and chopped
1 cup blackberries, fresh or frozen
¼ cup packed light brown sugar

Cook the apples and blackberries in a saucepan with the sugar and 2 tablespoons of water. Cook until the apples are soft (15–20 minutes). Put the fruit through a food mill to make into a smooth purée.

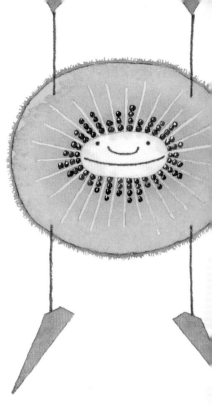

Apple and Raisin Rice Pudding ☺ ☹

Short-grain rice has a soft consistency, which is good for introducing texture into your baby's diet. It is great mixed with fruit purée like stewed apples and pears, or add some chopped dried fruit like apricots when you are cooking the rice.

MAKES 2 PORTIONS
2 tablespoons short-grain rice (such as Arborio rice)
1¼ cups whole milk
½ apple, peeled and grated
1 tablespoon golden raisins or dark raisins
1–2 teaspoons maple syrup

Put the rice and milk into a small saucepan. Bring to a boil, then cover and simmer over a gentle heat for 25–30 minutes, stirring from time to time, until the rice is cooked and the milk has reduced to a creamy consistency. Put the apple and raisins into a small pan with 3 tablespoons water. Simmer for a few minutes until the apple has softened. Stir into the rice, together with the maple syrup.

Fresh Fruit Ice Pops

Your baby will be teething at this age and, very often, sore gums can put her off eating for a while. Sucking on something cold soothes sore gums so a good idea is to make fresh fruit ice pops using puréed fruit, which you can mix with fruit juice or yogurt. You can even pour fruit smoothies or fresh juices straight into ice-pop molds.

Raspberry and Watermelon Ice Pops ❄ ☺ ☹

MAKES ABOUT 1½ CUPS OR 4 LARGE POPS
¼ watermelon
heaping ½ cup fresh raspberries
⅓–½ cup confectioner's sugar

Cut the flesh from the watermelon and remove the seeds. Blend the watermelon and raspberries together. Strain and stir in the confectioner's sugar to taste. Pour into ice-pop molds and freeze.

Tropical Ice Pops ❄ ☺ ☹

MAKES ABOUT 1½ CUPS OR 4 LARGE POPS
1 large mango, peeled, pitted, and diced
¾ cup tropical fruit juice
3 tablespoons confectioner's sugar
1 tablespoon lemon juice

Blend the ingredients together until smooth. Pour into ice-pop molds and freeze.

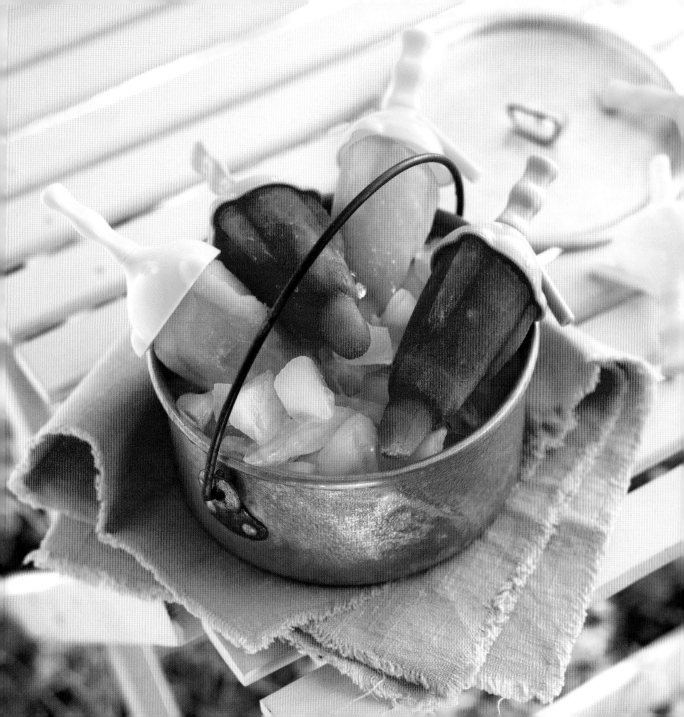

Yogurt Dip ☺ ☹

This yogurt dip is a great way to get your children to eat fruit. Try cutting up chunks of fruit such as strawberries, mango, or peach, or slices of apple, and using them to dip.

MAKES 1 PORTION

3 tablespoons Greek-style or regular plain yogurt
1 tablespoon seedless raspberry jam or jelly
1 teaspoon confectioners' sugar
½ teaspoon milk

Simply mix all the ingredients together. If you can only find jam with seeds, strain the dip after mixing, as children can find the small seeds unpalatable.

Dried Apricots with Papaya and Pear ❄ ☺ ☹

Dried apricots are rich in beta carotene and iron and they combine well with a variety of fresh fruits. This is also good mixed with yogurt. I found that my children also liked chewing on semi-dried apple rings, which are easy to hold because of the hole in the middle.

MAKES 4 PORTIONS

¼ cup ready-to-eat dried apricots, chopped
½ ripe papaya, peeled, seeded, and chopped
1 ripe juicy pear, peeled, cored, and chopped

Put the apricots into a small saucepan and just cover with water. Bring to a boil and simmer until softened (about 6–8 minutes). Mix the apricots with the papaya and pear, or purée for babies who prefer a smoother texture.

Vegetables

Risotto with Butternut Squash ❄ ☺ ☹

Cooked rice with vegetables is nice and soft so it's a good way to introduce texture to your baby's food. Butternut squash is now more readily available in supermarkets and it is rich in vitamin A. You could use pumpkin to make this, instead of squash.

MAKES 4 PORTIONS
½ cup onion, chopped
2 tablespoons butter
½ cup basmati rice
2 cups boiling water or vegetable broth
heaping ¾ cup butternut squash, peeled and diced
3 ripe tomatoes (about ½ lb), skinned, seeded, and chopped
½ cup Cheddar cheese, grated

Sauté the onion in half of the butter until softened. Stir in the rice until well coated. Pour over the boiling water or broth, cover, and cook for 8 minutes over a high heat. Stir in the butternut squash, reduce the heat, and cook, covered, for about 12 minutes or until the water has been absorbed.

Meanwhile, melt the remaining butter in a small saucepan, add the chopped tomatoes, and sauté for 2–3 minutes. Stir in the cheese until melted. Add the tomato and cheese mixture to the cooked rice and combine. Season to taste for babies over one year.

Lentil and Vegetable Purée ❄ ☺ ☹

This is one of my most popular purées. Lentils are a good, cheap source of protein. They also provide iron, which is very important for brain development, particularly between the ages of six months and two years.

A vegetarian baby's first tastes of food is the same as for other babies (baby rice, fruit, and vegetable purées, etc.). But, from around seven months when proteins are being introduced, instead of meat give foods like lentils, eggs, or dairy products.

It is not as easy to absorb iron from non-animal sources, so it's a good idea to give vitamin C–rich fruit or fruit juices as this helps to boost iron absorption.

MAKES 6 PORTIONS
1 tablespoon vegetable oil
½ cup chopped onion or leek (white part only)
1 cup peeled and chopped carrot
½ stalk chopped celery
¼ cup split red lentils
1½ cups peeled and chopped sweet potato
scant 1 cup tomato purée (no salt added)
½ cup grated sharp Cheddar cheese

Heat the vegetable oil and sauté the onion, carrot, and celery for 5 minutes. Rinse the lentils and add to the pan. Add the sweet potato and sauté for 1 minute. Pour in the tomato purée and 1 tablespoon water. Cover and cook for about 30 minutes. Remove from the heat and stir in the cheese until melted. Purée in a blender.

Multicolored Casserole ❄ ☺ ☹

Babies love the bright colors and miniature size of these vegetables. It makes eating fun, and is a good lesson in finger control.

MAKES 4 PORTIONS
1 tablespoon olive oil
1 shallot, peeled and finely chopped
½ oz red bell pepper, diced
1 cup frozen peas
1 cup frozen corn
½ cup vegetable broth (see page 38) or water

Heat the oil in a saucepan, add the shallot and bell pepper and cook for 3 minutes. Add the peas and corn, pour over the vegetable broth, and bring to a boil. Cover and simmer for 3–4 minutes.

Tasty Brown Rice ❄ ☺ ☹

Rice dishes are good for introducing more texture into your baby's food. You could also make this with white rice.

MAKES 6 PORTIONS
¼ cup brown rice
1 tablespoon vegetable oil
¾ cup carrot, peeled and grated
3 medium tomatoes, skinned, seeded, and chopped
⅓ cup Cheddar cheese, grated

Cook the rice in water following the instructions on the bag, until quite soft (about 30 minutes). Meanwhile, heat the oil in a pan, add the carrots, and sauté for 3 minutes. Add the tomatoes and cook for 2 more minutes. Drain the rice and mix with the carrot and tomatoes. Stir in the grated cheese and cook over a gentle heat for 1 minute until melted.

Vegetables in Cheese Sauce ❄ ☺ ☹

MAKES 6 PORTIONS

1 cup cauliflower florets
1 carrot, peeled and thinly sliced
½ cup frozen peas
1 cup zucchini, sliced

CHEESE SAUCE

2 tablespoons butter or margarine
2 tablespoons all-purpose flour
1 cup milk
½ cup Cheddar cheese, grated

Steam the cauliflower and carrot for 6 minutes, then add the peas and zucchini and cook for a further 4 minutes. For a young baby, cook the vegetables until they are soft.

Meanwhile, make the cheese sauce in the usual way (see page 67). Mash, chop, or purée the vegetables with the sauce.

Sweet Potato and Spinach Mash ☺☹

MAKES 3–4 PORTIONS

1 large sweet potato (3/4 lb)
1 large potato (1/2 lb)
1 medium carrot
2 cups baby spinach leaves, washed
a generous pat of butter
1 tablespoon milk
⅓ cup Cheddar cheese, grated

Peel and chop the sweet potato, potato, and carrot. Put them in a saucepan and just cover with boiling water. Cook until the vegetables are tender (around 15 minutes). Alternatively you can steam them. Drain the vegetables, add the spinach to the pan, and cook for 2 minutes. Mash the vegetables together with the butter, milk, and cheese.

Fish

Healthy Fish Sticks ☺☹

These little sticks of flounder are fun for babies and toddlers to eat, and make great finger food. They can be served plain or you can dip them into a homemade tomato sauce. Simply purée 3 peeled and seeded tomatoes with a sautéed shallot, 1 tablespoon tomato paste, 2 teaspoons milk, and a teaspoon of finely chopped fresh basil.

These fish sticks are much better for your child than commercial ones, which are full of coloring and additives. If you are not using all the fish sticks at once, it is best to freeze them before they are cooked. You can then take out as many as you need for a freshly cooked meal.

Crushed cornflakes also make a delicious coating for other types of fish like haddock or cod.

MAKES 8 PORTIONS
1 shallot, peeled and finely chopped
2 teaspoons lemon juice
1 tablespoon vegetable oil
1 flounder, filleted and skinned
1 egg
2 teaspoons milk
all-purpose flour
crushed cornflakes
a little butter or margarine for frying

Mix together the chopped shallot, lemon juice, and oil. Marinate the fish fillets in this mixture for 30 minutes. (If you're short of time, you could skip this stage.) Remove the fillets from the marinade. Cut them into 4 or 5 diagonal strips, depending on the size of the fish. Beat the egg together with the milk. Dip the strips first into the flour, then into the egg and milk, and finally into the crushed cornflakes. Fry the sticks in butter or margarine until golden brown on both sides. They should take no more than a few minutes to cook.

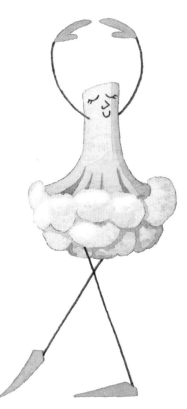

Salmon and Broccoli Pasta ❄ ☺ ☹

This recipe was sent to me by Kate Hanke, who lives in Oxford in the UK. She entered a competition that I ran together with Tumbletots, "Eat Fit, Keep Fit," to devise a recipe that would tempt fussy eaters. Kate's tip is to stay positive, try not to show concern about your child's eating habits, or describe your child as a "fussy eater" in front of her. If they believe they are good at eating a wide variety of healthy foods, they may well become good anyway. I found this recipe was quick, easy, and very tasty. Note: Unlike canned tuna, canned salmon does contain essential fatty acids.

MAKES 5 PORTIONS
¹/₂ lb animal pasta shapes
¹/₂ cup onion, finely chopped
1 garlic clove, crushed
a little butter or oil
2¹/₂ cups broccoli florets
1 x 3³/₄-oz can wild red salmon, drained and mashed
¹/₂ cup heavy cream
¹/₂ cup Parmesan cheese, grated
a little freshly ground black pepper

Cook the pasta following the box instructions. In a large pan, fry the onion and garlic in the butter or oil until soft (about 3–4 minutes). Steam the broccoli until tender (about 6 minutes). Add the cooked pasta to the onion. Add the salmon, cream, and broccoli and season with a little black pepper. Add the Parmesan cheese and mix well so that the cheese melts into the cream. Serve immediately.

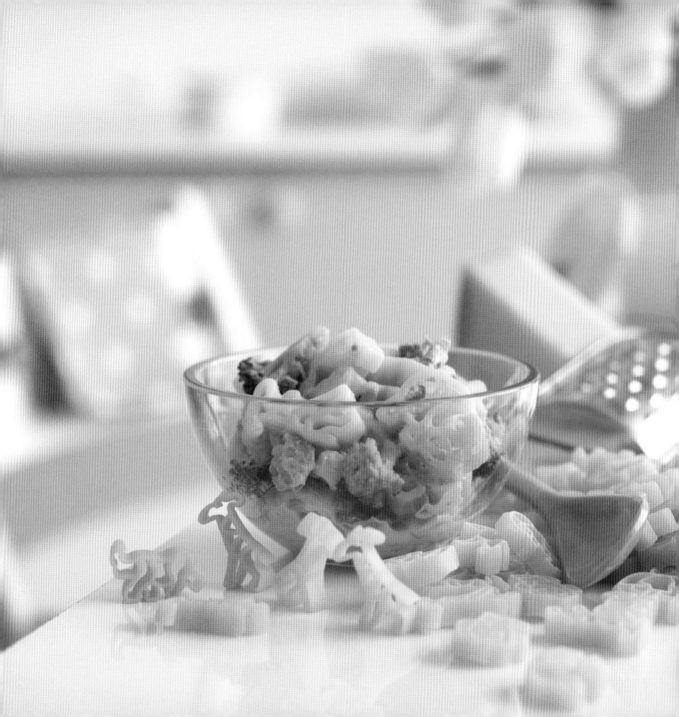

Fillets of Flounder with Grapes ❄ ☺ ☹

Fillets of flounder with grapes makes a delicious combination. This recipe is quick and easy to prepare and one that the whole family can enjoy.

MAKES 4 ADULT PORTIONS

8 small flounder fillets, skinned
salt and freshly ground black pepper (from one year)
2 tablespoons all-purpose flour
2 tablespoons butter
1 large or 2 small scallions, thinly sliced
1 teaspoon white wine vinegar
²/₃ cup fish broth
½ cup heavy cream
1 tablespoon snipped chives
½ cup seedless white grapes, halved or quartered if large
1–2 teaspoons lemon juice (to taste)

Season the fish with a little salt and pepper (if using) and dust with flour. Heat a large frying pan and add the butter. When the butter is foaming, add the fish and cook over medium-high heat for about 2 minutes on each side, until the fish is golden and cooked through. Transfer to a plate and keep warm. You may need to cook the fillets in two batches, in which case use half the butter for each batch.

Reduce the heat to low, add the scallion, and cook for 1 minute, then add the vinegar and cook until evaporated. Add the broth, bring to a boil, and cook for 2 minutes until reduced by half. Stir in the cream, chives, and grapes and remove from the heat. Add 1 teaspoon lemon juice and season to taste, adding extra lemon if needed. Spoon the sauce over the fish to serve.

Baked Fish in a Package ☺ ☹

Fish is easy to cook. You can cook it very quickly in the microwave, but here
I have wrapped it in parchment paper and baked it in the oven.

MAKES 2 PORTIONS
a little olive oil for greasing
2 skinless fillets of flounder
a little salt and freshly ground black pepper (from one year)
½ teaspoon finely snipped chives
1 slice lemon
a pat of butter
1 fat scallion, thinly sliced
1 tablespoon frozen peas
2 tablespoons crème fraîche or heavy cream
1–2 teaspoons milk (optional)
2 teaspoons grated Parmesan cheese (optional)

Preheat the oven to 400°F. Lightly grease a piece of parchment paper with oil
and put the fish in the center. Season with a little salt and pepper (if using) and
sprinkle with the chives. Lay the slice of lemon on the fish and fold the parchment
to form a package (fastened with paper clips if necessary). Bake for 8 minutes, or
until the fish is tender.

Meanwhile, melt the butter in a small saucepan and sauté the scallion for
1–2 minutes, until soft. Add the peas and cook for 1 minute, then add the crème
fraîche or cream and cook, stirring, for 1–2 minutes, until the peas are cooked.
Remove from the heat.

Open up the parchment and discard the lemon. Transfer the fish to a plate and
pour the remaining juices into the saucepan. Stir the sauce and add 1–2 teaspoons
of milk, if needed, to make it slightly thinner. Season to taste with salt and pepper
(from one year).

For smaller babies, the fish, peas, and sauce can be mashed or
puréed. Also, stir 2 teaspoons grated Parmesan into the sauce
instead of seasoning with salt and pepper.

Serve with rice or boiled baby potatoes.

Salmon Footballs ❄ ☺ ☹

These nutritious finger foods are ideal when your child refuses to eat anything from a spoon. Omit the salt and pepper for babies under one year.

MAKES 10 SMALL FOOTBALLS

1 medium white potato such as Yukon, skin on
3 oz salmon fillet
a squeeze of lemon juice
a pat of butter
2 scallions, chopped
1 teaspoon sweet chili sauce (optional)
2 tablespoons tomato ketchup
½ tablespoon mayonnaise
salt and freshly ground black pepper (from one year)
1 tablespoon seasoned all-purpose flour
1 egg, lightly beaten
heaping ⅓ cup dried breadcrumbs
canola oil for frying

DIP

3 tablespoons mayonnaise
½ teaspoon sweet chili sauce

Boil the potato in salted water for 25–30 minutes until tender when pierced with a table knife. Drain and, when cool enough to handle, peel and mash.

Cook the salmon in the microwave on High for 2–3 minutes with the lemon juice and butter. Flake the flesh onto a plate and leave to cool slightly. Mix the potato with the scallions, chili sauce (if using), tomato ketchup, mayonnaise, and salt and pepper to taste. Fold in the flaked salmon, taking care not to break up the fish too much.

Take 1½ tablespoons of the mixture and form into a ball. Repeat until you have used up all the mixture. Dust each ball in the flour, dip in the egg, then roll in the breadcrumbs. Heat some canola oil in a non-stick pan and deep-fry the footballs for 2–3 minutes. You can shallow fry the footballs in 2 tablespoons of oil but they won't keep their round shape so well. Cool slightly before serving.

To make the dip, mix together the mayonnaise and sweet chili sauce.

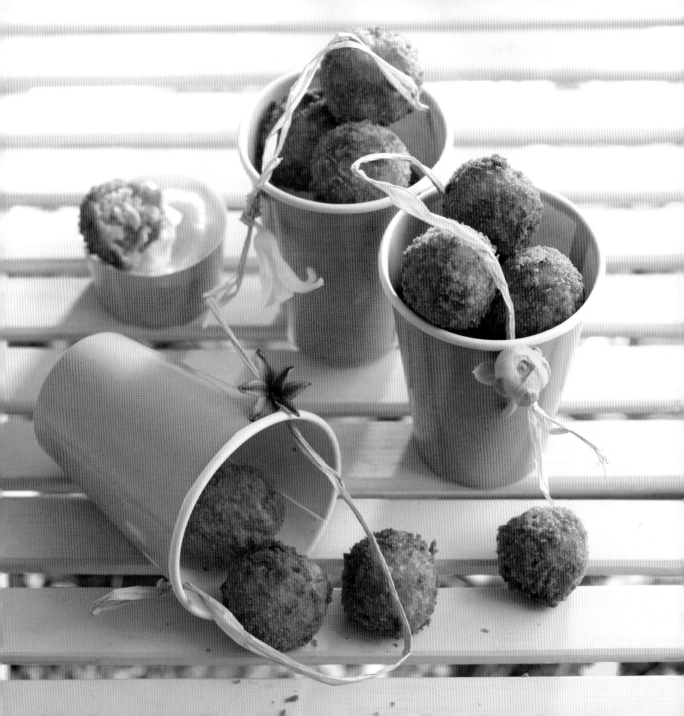

Chicken

Chicken and Apple Balls ❄ ☺ ☹

This is a great favorite with my family. Grated apple adds a delicious flavor to these chicken balls, which makes them appealing to young children, and they are delicious hot or cold. These little balls make perfect finger food.

MAKES 20 CHICKEN BALLS
2 teaspoons light olive oil
1 onion, finely chopped
1 large Granny Smith apple, peeled and grated
2 chicken breast fillets (about ½ lb), cut into chunks
½ tablespoon fresh parsley, chopped
1 tablespoon fresh thyme or sage, chopped, or a pinch mixed dried herbs
1 chicken bouillon cube, crumbled (from one year)
1 cup fresh white breadcrumbs
salt and freshly ground pepper (from one year)
all-purpose flour for coating
vegetable oil for frying

Heat the olive oil in a pan and sauté half the onion for about 3 minutes. Using your hands, squeeze out a little excess liquid from the grated apple. Mix the apple with the chicken, cooked and remaining raw onion, herbs, bouillon cube (from one year), and breadcrumbs and roughly chop in a food processor for a few seconds. Season with a little salt and pepper (from one year).

With your hands, form into about 20 little balls, roll in flour, and fry in shallow oil for about 5 minutes until lightly golden and cooked through. Cool slightly before serving.

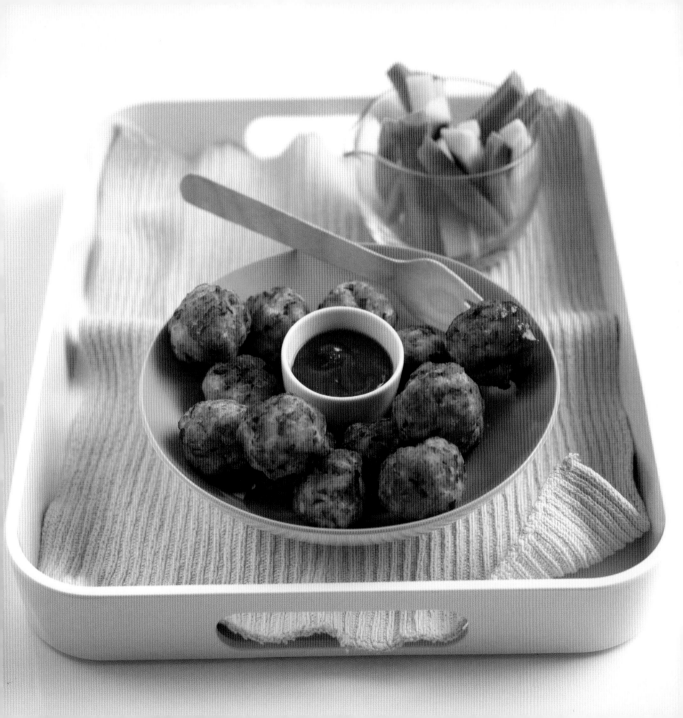

Bang Bang Chicken ❄ ☺ ☹

So called because my son liked to help flatten the chicken by banging it with a mallet! If you want to prepare these chicken strips in advance, wrap each strip separately (before frying) and freeze. Just take one or two strips out of the freezer and fry them for freshly cooked chicken fingers.

MAKES 8 PORTIONS
2 chicken breast fillets (about ½ lb)
3 slices bread, crusts removed
1½ tablespoons Parmesan cheese, grated (optional)
1 tablespoon fresh parsley, chopped (optional)
plain flour for coating
1 egg, beaten
vegetable oil

Cover the chicken with parchment or wax paper and flatten with a mallet or rolling pin, then cut each breast lengthways into four strips. Make breadcrumbs from the slices of bread in a food processor. If you are using the Parmesan and parsley, mix these together with the breadcrumbs in a bowl.

Dip the chicken into the flour, then into the egg, and then finally into the breadcrumbs. Fry in oil for 3–4 minutes each side until golden on the outside and cooked through. Drain on absorbent kitchen paper, cool slightly, and serve.

Chicken with Cornflakes ❄ ☺ ☹

Cornflakes are very versatile and I often use them instead of breadcrumbs to coat both chicken and fish. These strips of chicken make good finger food. Before cooking, they can be individually wrapped and frozen.

MAKES 3–4 PORTIONS
1 egg, beaten
1 tablespoon milk
1 cup cornflakes, crushed
1 large chicken breast fillet cut into about 8 strips
1 tablespoon butter, melted

Mix together the egg and milk in a shallow dish. In a separate dish spread out the cornflake crumbs. Dip the strips of chicken into the egg and then coat with the cornflakes. Put the chicken strips into a greased ovenproof dish, drizzle over the melted butter, and toss to coat. Bake in an oven preheated to 350°F for about 10 minutes on each side, or until cooked through. Alternatively, the chicken strips can be sautéed in vegetable oil until golden and cooked through. Cool slightly before serving.

Chicken with Summer Vegetables ❄ ☺ ☹

The sweet potato, apple juice, and peas add a natural sweetness that babies like. The garlic and basil adds flavor, which is important since you can't add salt before one year of age.

MAKES 5 PORTIONS

1 small onion, chopped
½ small red bell pepper, seeded and finely chopped
1½ tablespoons olive oil
1 garlic clove, crushed
1 chicken breast fillet (about ¼ lb), cut into pieces
2 tablespoons apple juice
⅔ cup chicken broth (see page 76)
1 medium zucchini, chopped
1½ cups sweet potato, peeled and diced
½ cup frozen peas
1 tablespoon fresh basil, torn

Sauté the onion and bell pepper in the olive oil until softened. Add the garlic and sauté for 1 minute. Stir in the chicken and continue to cook for 3–4 minutes. Pour over the apple juice and broth and stir in the zucchini, and sweet potato. Bring to a boil, then cover and simmer for about 8 minutes. Stir in the peas and continue to cook for 3 minutes. Chop or pureé to the desired consistency.

Chicken with Winter Vegetables ❄ ☺ ☹

This is quick and easy to prepare and has a delicious rich chicken flavor.

MAKES 6 PORTIONS
1 chicken breast portion (about 6 oz), on the bone and skinned
a little all-purpose flour
vegetable oil
1 leek, white part only, washed and sliced
1 small onion, peeled and finely chopped
3 carrots, peeled and sliced
1 celery stalk, trimmed and sliced
1²/₃ cups chicken broth (see page 76)

Cut the chicken breast in half, roll each half in flour, and brown in a little oil for 3–4 minutes. In another skillet, sauté the leek and onion in a little oil for 5 minutes until soft and golden. Put the chicken into a Dutch oven together with all the vegetables and the broth. Cook in an oven preheated to 350°F for 1 hour, stirring halfway through.

Take the chicken off the bone and chop it into little pieces with the vegetables or purée it together with the cooking liquid in a food mill or blender.

Chicken with Couscous ❄ ☺ ☹

MAKES 4 PORTIONS
1 tablespoon butter
2 tablespoons onion, chopped
¹/₄ cup frozen peas (cooked)
²/₃ cup chicken broth (see page 76)
¹/₃ cup quick-cook couscous
¹/₄ cup chicken, cooked and diced

Melt the butter in a saucepan and sauté the onion until softened but not colored. Stir in the peas, pour over the broth, bring to the boil, and cook for 3 minutes. Stir in the couscous, remove from the heat, cover, and set aside for 6 minutes. Fluff the couscous with a fork and mix in the diced chicken.

Red meats

Beef Casserole with Carrots ❄ ☺ ☹

The secret for a delicious rich taste is to cook the meat for a long time so that it is very tender and has a good flavor from the onions and carrots.

MAKES 10 PORTIONS
2 medium onions, peeled and sliced
vegetable oil
3/4 lb lean stewing beef, trimmed and cut into small chunks
2 medium carrots, peeled and sliced
1 beef bouillon cube, crumbled (for babies over one year)
1 tablespoon fresh parsley, chopped
2 1/2 cups water
2 large potatoes, peeled and cut into quarters

Fry the onion in a little oil until golden, then add the meat chunks and brown. Transfer the meat and onions to a small Dutch oven and add the remaining ingredients except for the potatoes. Cook, covered, in an oven preheated to 350°F for 30 minutes, then turn down the heat and cook for a further 2½ hours at 325°F. An hour before you finish cooking the meat, add the potatoes.

Chop the casserole quite finely in a food processor or blender so that it is easy for your baby to chew. If the meat gets too dry whilst cooking, add a little extra water. For variation, you can also add sliced mushrooms and diced tomatoes to this recipe 30 minutes before the end of cooking time.

Tasty Liver Casserole ❄ ☺ ☹

Liver is very good for children: it is easy to digest, a good source of iron, and is very easy to cook. I must admit that I dislike the taste, having been forced to eat liver at school, but, to my great surprise, my one-year-old son adored it. This recipe is good served with mashed potato.

MAKES 4 PORTIONS
¼ lb calf's liver, trimmed and sliced
2 tablespoons vegetable oil
1 small onion, peeled and chopped
1 large or 2 medium carrots (about ¼ lb), peeled and chopped
scant 1 cup chicken or vegetable broth (see pages 76 and 38)
2 medium tomatoes (about ½ lb), skinned, seeded, and chopped
2 teaspoons fresh parsley, chopped

Sauté the liver in 1 tablespoon of the oil until browned, then set aside. Heat the remaining oil in a saucepan and sauté the onion for 2–3 minutes. Add the chopped carrot and sauté for 2 minutes, then pour in the broth, bring to a boil, cover, and simmer over low heat for about 15 minutes. Chop the liver into pieces and add to the pan together with the tomatoes and parsley, and cook for about 3 minutes. You can either serve with mashed potatoes as it is or blend the mixture for a few seconds to make a rough purée.

Savory Veal Casserole ❄ ☺ ☹

A delicious casserole of veal, vegetables, and fresh herbs – just increase the quantities for a meal the whole family can enjoy.

MAKES 3 PORTIONS
1 tablespoon vegetable or canola oil
1 large onion, peeled and finely chopped
1 large carrot, peeled and diced
½ celery stalk, diced
⅓ cup peeled, diced butternut squash

¼ lb lean veal for stewing, cut into chunks
1 sprig fresh rosemary
1 sprig fresh parsley
scant 1 cup water or unsalted chicken broth (see page 76)

Heat the oil. Add the onion, carrot, and celery and fry for 3–4 minutes. Add the squash and veal and fry for another 4 minutes. Add the herbs and water or broth. Bring to a boil, cover with a lid, and gently simmer for 1 hour. Remove the herbs, then coarsely chop in a food processor.

Special Steak ❄ ☺ ☹

This recipe makes a very good introduction to red meat for your baby.

MAKES 4 PORTIONS
1 potato (about ½ lb), peeled and diced
1 shallot or ¼ of an onion, peeled and finely chopped
1 tablespoon vegetable oil
¼ lb filet mignon or beef tenderloin
⅔ cup washed and chopped button mushrooms
1 tablespoon butter
1 tomato, skinned, seeded, and chopped
2 tablespoons milk

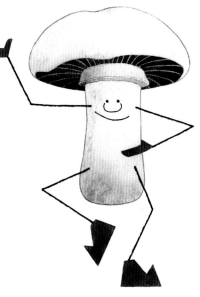

Boil the potato until tender, then drain. Meanwhile, sauté the shallot in the vegetable oil until softened. Spoon half the shallot onto a piece of aluminum foil. Cut the steak into slices ½ inch thick and place on top of the shallot. Spread the remaining shallot over the steak. Cook under a preheated broiler for 3 minutes each side or until cooked. Sauté the mushrooms in half of the butter for 2 minutes, add the chopped tomato, and continue to cook for 1 minute. Mash the potato with the milk and the remaining butter until smooth. Chop or purée the steak together with the shallots, mushrooms, and tomato and mix with the mashed potato.

Mini Cottage Pie ❄ ☺ ☹

Cottage pie was always popular as "comfort food" on a winter's evening when I was a child. To make it suitable for babies, I have chopped the meat in a food processor to make it softer. For babies over one you can season with a little salt and pepper. Try making individual portions in ramekin dishes. You can pop the extra portions in the freezer for days when you don't have time to cook.

MAKES 3 PORTIONS

1 cup carrot, peeled and chopped
2 cups potato, peeled and diced
1 tablespoon olive oil
1 small onion, peeled and chopped
¼ red bell pepper cored, seeded, and diced
1 small garlic clove, peeled and crushed
6 oz lean ground beef
1 tablespoon freshly chopped parsley
2 teaspoons tomato paste
scant ½ cup chicken broth (see page 76)
1 tablespoon butter
1 tablespoon milk
1 egg, beaten

Put the carrot into a saucepan, cover with boiling water, and cook for 5 minutes. Add the potato and cook for a further 15 minutes.

Meanwhile, heat the oil in a skillet, and sauté the onion and bell pepper for 3 to 4 minutes. Add the garlic and sauté for 1 minute. Add the ground beef and sauté until browned. At this stage it is a good idea to chop the meat in a food processor for a few seconds to give it a smoother texture. Return to the pan, add the parsley, tomato paste, and chicken broth, bring to a boil, then cover and simmer for about 5 minutes. When the potato and carrot are cooked, strain and mash with the butter and milk.

Spoon the meat into 3 ramekins about 4 inches in diameter. Top with the mashed potato and carrot. Brush with a little beaten egg, then heat through in an oven preheated to 350°F, then place under a preheated broiler until lightly golden.

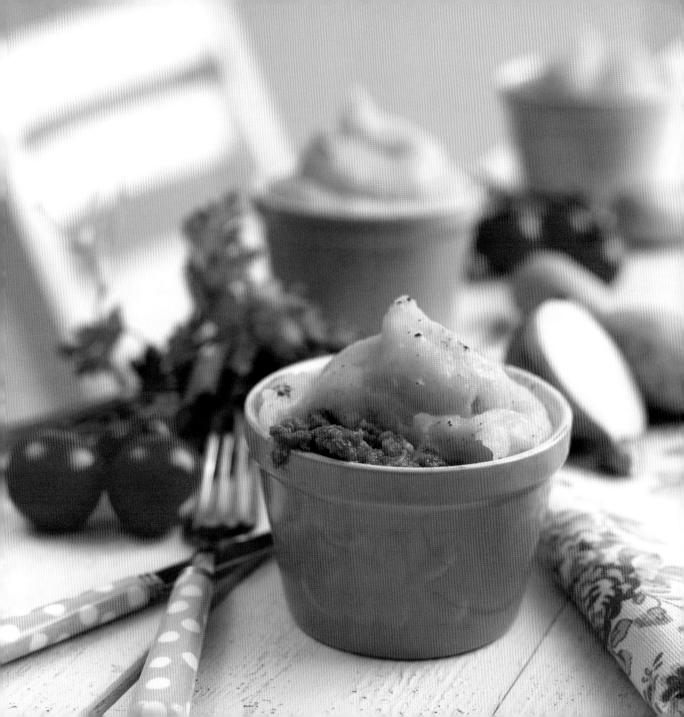

Tasty Rice with Meat and Vegetables ❄ ☺ ☹

MAKES 8 PORTIONS

⅓ cup basmati rice
1 tablespoon vegetable oil
1 medium red onion, peeled and finely chopped
1 carrot, peeled and finely chopped
½ eating apple, peeled and grated
1 small garlic clove, crushed
½ lb lean ground beef
1 x 14-oz can diced tomatoes
½ cup chicken broth (see page 76)
2 tablespoons apple juice
1 tablespoon tomato ketchup
a few drops of Worcestershire sauce, such as Lea and Perrins
¼ teaspoon mixed dried herbs
½ cup frozen peas

Rinse the rice and place in a saucepan with water or chicken broth, following the instructions on the bag.

Meanwhile, heat the oil in a pan and sauté the onion, carrot, and apple for 5 minutes. Add the garlic and sauté for 1 minute. Add the ground meat and cook, stirring, until browned. Add the chopped tomatoes, broth, apple juice, tomato ketchup, Worcestershire sauce, and herbs, and cook over a low heat uncovered for 20 minutes. You may wish to transfer the meat to a food processor and chop for 30 seconds to make it easier for your baby to chew. Return the meat to the pan, add the peas, and continue to cook for 3 minutes. Finally, stir in the rice.

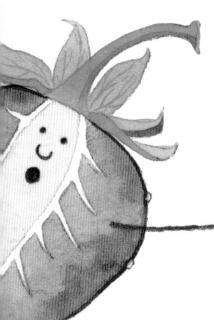
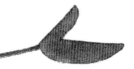

Pasta

Pasta-Shell Confetti ❋ ☺ ☹

There are many types of tiny pasta shapes available, such as mini pasta shells and novelty pasta like animals and alphabet shapes. Pasta-Shell Confetti can be mixed with lots of different vegetables – peas and broccoli would make a good combination.

MAKES 2–3 PORTIONS
1 tablespoon butter
⅓ cup carrot, peeled and diced
⅓ cup zucchini, diced
1 medium tomato, skinned, seeded, and chopped
½ cup tiny pasta shapes
3 tablespoons heavy cream
¼ cup Parmesan cheese, grated

Melt the butter and sauté the carrot for 3 minutes. Add the zucchini and cook gently for 8 minutes. Add the tomato and cook for 1 more minute.

Cook the pasta in plenty of boiling water following the box instructions. Drain the pasta and stir into the vegetables. Remove from the heat and stir in the cream and Parmesan cheese.

Bolognese Sauce with Eggplant ❄ ☺ ☹

MAKES 12 PORTIONS OF SAUCE

1 medium onion, peeled and chopped
¼ garlic clove, peeled and chopped
vegetable oil for frying
1 lb lean ground beef or lamb
2 tablespoons tomato paste
4 tomatoes, skinned, seeded, and chopped
¼ teaspoon mixed dried herbs
2 tablespoons all-purpose flour
scant 2 cups chicken broth (see page 76)
1 eggplant, peeled and sliced
1¼ cups cremini mushrooms, washed and sliced

Sauté the onion and garlic in oil until soft. Add the meat and cook until browned.
Chop in a food processor. Return to the pan, add the tomato paste, tomatoes, herbs,
flour, and broth. Bring to a boil and simmer for 45 minutes. Fry the eggplant in oil
until golden. Pat dry with kitchen paper. Chop in a food processor. Sauté the
mushrooms in oil and add to the sauce with the eggplant.

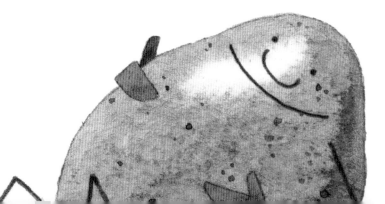

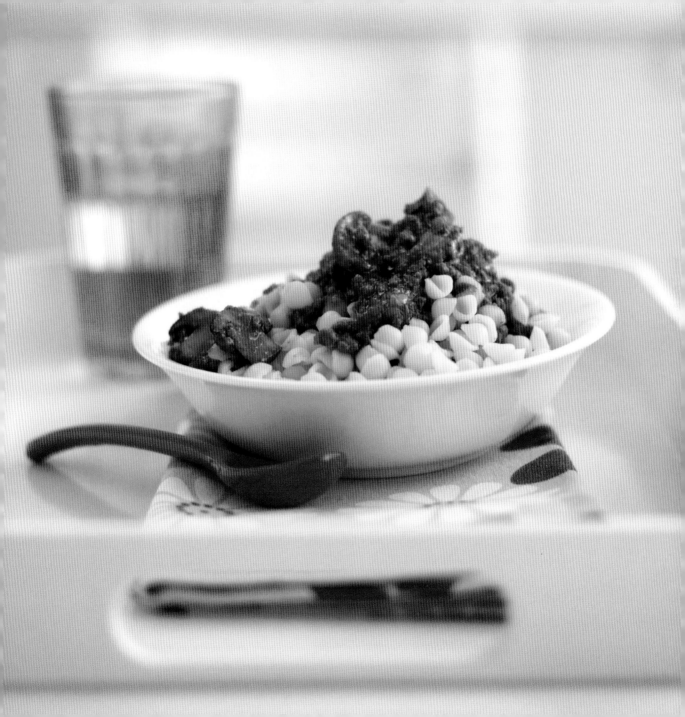

Pasta Shells with Hidden-Vegetable Bolognese ❄ ☺ ☹

A tasty tomato-based sauce with five vegetables blended in.

MAKES 8 PORTIONS

2 tablespoons olive oil

1 small red onion, finely chopped

1 small leek, finely sliced

3 mushrooms, sliced

1 carrot, grated

1 stalk celery, diced

1 garlic clove, crushed

$^2/_3$ cup beef or chicken broth (see page 76)

9 oz ground beef

2 x 14-oz cans diced tomatoes

3 tablespoons tomato paste

1 tablespoon tomato ketchup

$^1/_2$ lb mini pasta shells

Heat 1 tablespoon of the olive oil in a pan and sauté the onion for 3 minutes. Add the leek, mushrooms, carrot, and celery and sauté for 7 minutes. Add the garlic and sauté for 1 minute. Add half of the broth and simmer for 10 minutes, then put in a food processor and blitz. Heat the remaining tablespoon of olive oil in a large skillet and brown the ground beef for 5 minutes, breaking up well with a fork or wooden spoon. Add the canned tomatoes, tomato paste, tomato ketchup, and the remaining broth, and cook for 10 minutes. Add the blended vegetables and continue to cook for 2 minutes.

Meanwhile, cook the pasta following the box instructions. Drain and toss with the sauce.

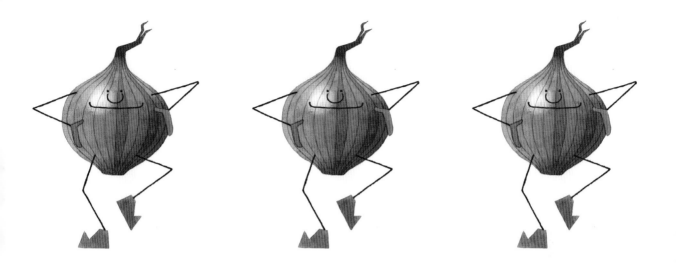

Pasta Shells with Chicken and Broccoli ❋ ☺ ☹

MAKES 2 PORTIONS
½ cup broccoli florets
1 tablespoon butter
1 tablespoon flour
⅔ cup milk
⅓ cup Gruyère cheese, grated
3 tablespoons Parmesan cheese, grated
3 tablespoons mascarpone cheese
⅓ cup pasta shells
¼ cup cooked chicken, diced

Steam the broccoli for 4–5 minutes or until tender. Melt the butter, stir in the flour, and cook for 1 minute. Gradually add the milk, then continue to stir for 5 minutes over a low heat until the sauce thickens. Take off the heat, stir in the Gruyère and Parmesan until melted, then stir in the mascarpone.

Meanwhile, cook the pasta following the box instructions. Drain and toss with the broccoli, chicken, and cheese sauce.

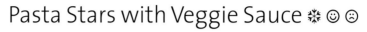

Pasta Stars with Veggie Sauce ❄ ☺ ☹

This fresh tomato sauce is very tasty and, because it has vegetables and cheese blended into it, it is more nutritious than an ordinary tomato sauce.

MAKES 2 PORTIONS
1 medium carrot, peeled and sliced
1 cup cauliflower florets
3 tablespoons pasta stars or other tiny pasta shapes
2 tablespoons butter
3/4 lb ripe tomatoes, skinned, seeded, and chopped
1/2 cup Cheddar cheese, grated

Put the sliced carrot into the bottom of a steamer. Cover with boiling water and cook over a medium heat for 10 minutes. Put the cauliflower florets in the steamer basket, place over the carrots, cover, and cook for 5 minutes or until the vegetables are tender. Cook the pasta stars in boiling water following the box instructions. Meanwhile, melt the butter and sauté the tomatoes for about 3 minutes or until mushy. Stir in the Cheddar cheese until melted. Blend the cooked carrots and cauliflower together with the tomatoes and cheese. Mix with the pasta stars.

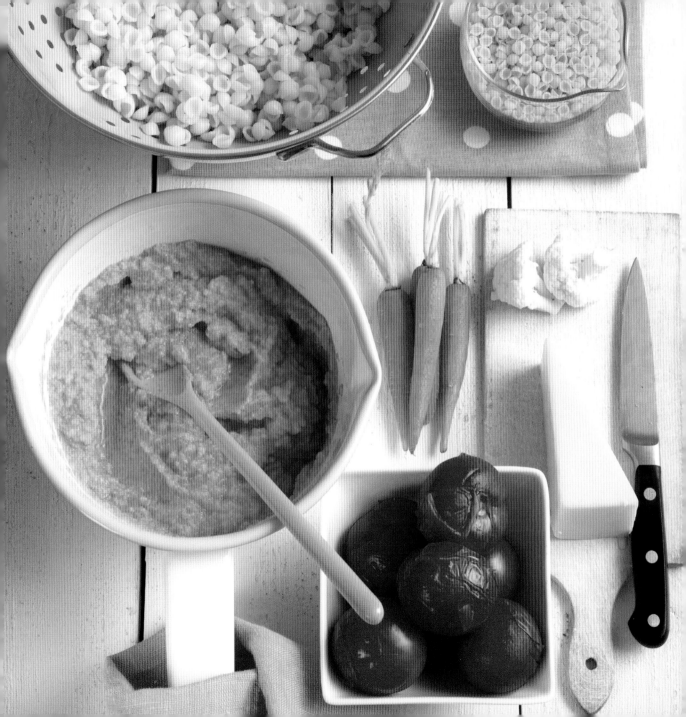

Nine to twelve month meal planner

	Breakfast	Mid-morning	Lunch	Mid-afternoon	Dinner	Bedtime
Day 1	**Fruity Swiss Muesli** **Dried Apricots with Papaya and Pear** served with yogurt Milk	Milk	**Chicken and Apple Balls** Vegetable sticks **Fresh Fruit with Yogurt Dip** Water	Milk	Finger sandwiches Vegetable sticks Juice or water	Milk
Day 2	Cheerios Broiled cheese on toast Fruit Milk	Milk	**Special Steak** **Apple and Raisin Rice Pudding** Water	Milk	**Pasta Stars with Veggie Sauce** Yogurt Juice or water	Milk
Day 3	Scrambled egg with toast Fruit with cottage cheese Milk	Milk	**Salmon Footballs** **Fresh Fruit Ice Pops** Water	Milk	**Tasty Brown Rice** Fruit Juice or water	Milk
Day 4	**My Favorite Crêpes** Fruit Milk	Milk	**Mini Cottage Pie** Fruit Water	Milk	**Vegetables in Cheese Sauce** **Apple and Blackberry** Juice or water	Milk

	Breakfast	Mid-morning	Lunch	Mid-afternoon	Dinner	Bedtime
Day 5	**French Toast Cutouts** **Apricot, Apple, and Pear Custard** Milk	Milk	**Bang Bang Chicken** **Tasty Brown Rice** **Fresh Fruit with Yogurt Dip** Water	Milk	**Risotto and Butternut Squash** Fruit Juice or water	Milk
Day 6	**Summer Fruit Muesli** Yogurt with dried fruit Milk	Milk	**Pasta Shells with Hidden-Vegetable Bolognese** **Apple and Blackberry** Water	Milk	**Healthy Fish Sticks** Vegetable sticks **Fresh Fruit Ice Pops** Juice or water	Milk
Day 7	**Cheese Scramble** Toast sticks Yogurt Milk	Milk	**Chicken with Couscous** **Fresh Fruit with Yogurt Dip** Water	Milk	**Lentil and Vegetable Purée** Sticks of cheese **Baked Apples with Raisins** Juice or water	Milk

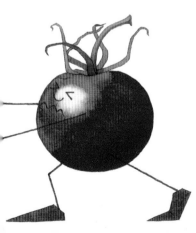

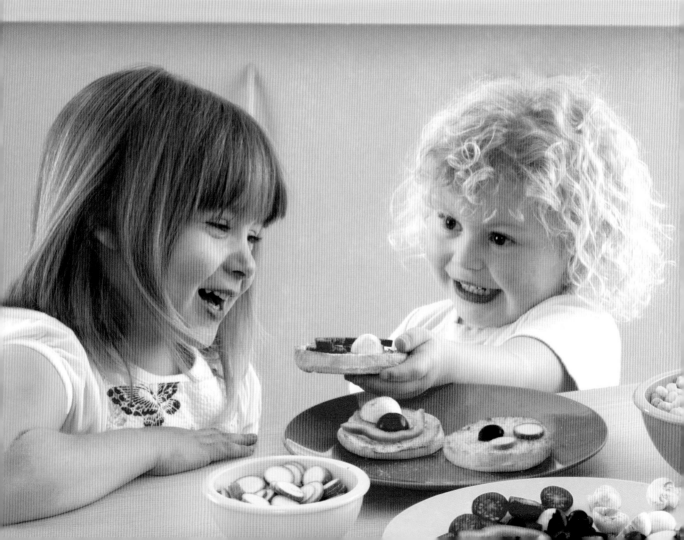

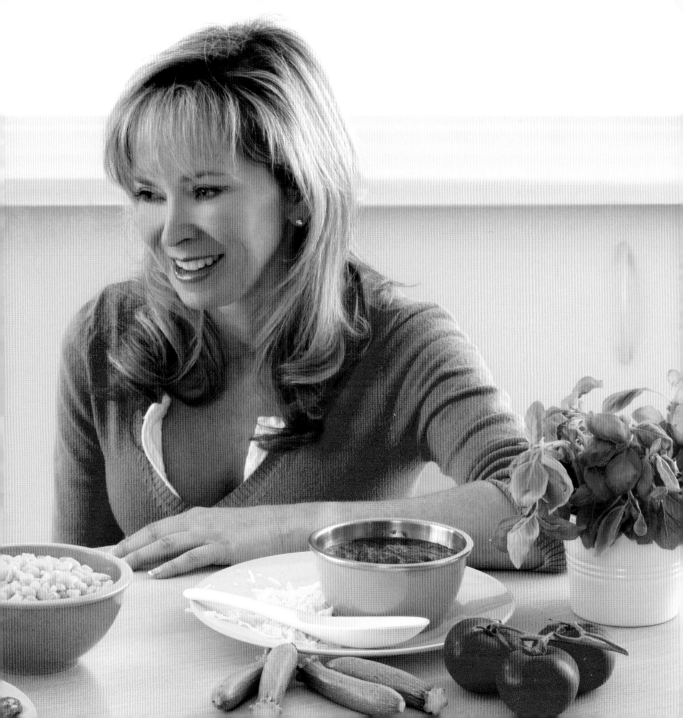

I find that, beyond the age of one, toddlers prefer to exercise their independence and feed themselves. The more your toddler experiments using a spoon and fork, the quicker he will master the art of feeding himself – you never know, some food might find its way into his mouth! A "pelican" bib – a strong plastic bib which has a tray at the bottom to catch stray food – is also good. If your toddler has difficulty eating with a spoon, try giving him finger foods like goujons of fish or raw vegetables with a dip. You must still be careful, though, to keep food like olives, nuts, or fresh lychees out of the reach of young children. Toddlers love to put everything in their mouths and it would be so easy for them to choke on such foods.

Enjoying mealtimes together

Toddlers only have small tummies and often can't eat enough at mealtimes to fuel their high energy requirements, so they should be offered three meals and snacks at regular times. It's a good idea to have a shelf in your refrigerator with some healthy snacks like raw vegetables and a dip, e.g. hummus, sticks of cheese, and a variety of fresh fruit. For more ideas for healthy snacks, take a look at my book *After-School Meal Planner*. Toddlers who get used to eating healthy snacks are more likely to continue the same habits later on in life. However, it would also be wrong to make sweets and chocolate biscuits the forbidden fruit, as your toddler would crave them all the more and gorge himself on them whenever he could.

Many toddlers enjoy eating much more sophisticated food than we would imagine. My daughter at two loved cut-up olives, for example. Ethnic recipes like stir-fries with noodles or egg-fried rice with chicken tend to be popular, and you can buy child-friendly chopsticks that are joined at the top and make eating fun. Dump the chicken dinosaurs coated in bread crumbs and marinate chicken to make recipes like my Thai-style Chicken and Noodles or Chicken Satay (see pages 170 and 172). Even if you don't feel like making your own marinade, there are lots of delicious marinades available in the ethnic foods section of the supermarket that will spice up your child's food. Let your child try food from your plate and you may be very surprised by the tastes he enjoys. Of course, food from Mommy's or Daddy's plate is much more interesting than his own meal, and you can sometimes entice your child to eat if you put his meal on your plate. But the point at this stage is that the toddler can now eat, to a large extent, what you adults are eating. I am a great believer in giving toddlers "grown-up" foods as soon as possible, and almost all the recipes that follow are suitable for the whole family. Do eat with your child rather than just sitting there shoveling food into his mouth. He'll eat much more happily with you – after all, who enjoys eating alone?

Try to reform your own eating habits by adding less salt and sugar to your food and get your child to help plan, shop for, and cook a meal. Obviously you can't do this every day but, if you do it every so often, it's a good way of introducing new meals to your child.

My child won't eat!

Anyone with a fussy child will know that it's easy to lose heart when your child turns his nose up at anything with visible onions or tomato sauce with green bits in it. I think the key to success is not to get into a tizzy if your child doesn't eat – just say "fine," but don't offer anything else until the next meal. Refusing food loses its appeal if you don't react, and it's amazing how much less fussy your child will become if he is really hungry. I would ignore any negative behavior and pile on the praise when your child does try something – even if the tiniest morsel passes his lips, go overboard with praise. A star chart might be a good idea, where your child gets a star for any new food or recipe that he tries. When he collects a certain number of stars, he gets a reward.

Rest assured that if you have a fussy toddler you are not alone. Toddlers can thrive very well on remarkably little food. They are also unpredictable – one day they can like something and the next day they refuse to eat it. Some days they will be ravenous and other days they will eat practically nothing. If you monitor your child's food intake over a whole week, you won't worry as much if one day he refuses to eat anything.

Often it's snacks between meals that spoil your child's appetite. Try to resist buying chocolate cookies and chips and instead offer healthy alternatives like mini-sandwiches, chopped dried fruit, or even a bowl of healthy cereal.

Be sure your child isn't filling up on drinks. What he drinks can have a huge effect on his appetite. Give juice or smoothies that are 100 percent juice instead of fruit juice drinks, which often contain less than 10 percent juice and can contain artificial sweeteners, flavorings, and colorings, as well as added sugar – some with more than six teaspoons of sugar in a glass. Tap water is the best way to quench your thirst, and it's safe, cheap, and calorie-free.

A gift wrapped in bright paper with a beautiful ribbon inspires more enthusiasm than one given in a brown cardboard box, and the same goes for food that we serve our kids. You can transform a plain-Jane peanut butter sandwich into an irresistible kids' treat when it's cut into a heart or a teddy bear shape. Instead of whole fruit in a fruit bowl, thread bite-sized pieces of fruit onto a skewer or straw, or purée fruit and freeze it in ice-pop molds.

Don't put too much food on a plate – much better that your child should ask for more. Toddlers love individual portions of food and it's good to make mini portions of larger pies.

Getting children to try a new food is not easy – of my three children, two were quite fussy so I've tried all the tricks myself. Inviting a child over for tea who is a good eater is an excellent ruse. At all costs avoid confrontation – it's much better to turn "weird" food into a game by blindfolding your child and then asking him to try a selection of foods, some familiar and some new, and then guess what they are . . .

If you enjoy the recipes in this chapter, look out for my sequel to this book, *Favorite Family Meals*.

The foods to choose

Children under five need more dietary fat than adults in proportion to their body weight, so unless your child is overweight, don't give him foods that are low-fat. Fats like cheese or full-fat yogurt are a rich source of energy which your toddler needs to fuel his growth. There are, of course, exceptions to the rule, and an overweight toddler should have his fat intake restricted by cutting down on processed and fatty foods and switching to low-fat dairy products.

High-fiber foods in large amounts are also unsuitable as they are bulky and filling and do not supply enough calories for a rapidly growing toddler. Also, a high-fiber diet can hinder the absorption of vital minerals like iron. Provided your child eats plenty of fruit and vegetables, he will get all the fiber he needs.

Once your child is twelve months old you can switch from infant formula to whole cow's milk, but don't give reduced-fat or low-fat milk before the age of two as it is low in calories, which your child needs to grow. Fat-free milk should not be introduced before five years. Children over one year need 14 oz 1²/3 cups) of whole milk a day. For children who are very picky, there may be advantages to continuing with a follow-on formula (which is fortified with vitamins and iron) until two years of age.

Although more and more people seem to be turning away from red meat in favor of fish and chicken, bear in mind that red meat provides more iron and zinc than either fish or poultry. Try making tasty meals with lean ground meat – a good tip is to cook the meat and then chop it in a food processor so that it is not lumpy, and there are some lovely recipes for Beefburgers, Meatballs and Mini Minute Steaks (see pages 178–81) that make excellent family meals. Try to avoid processed meats like sausages, salami, and corned beef.

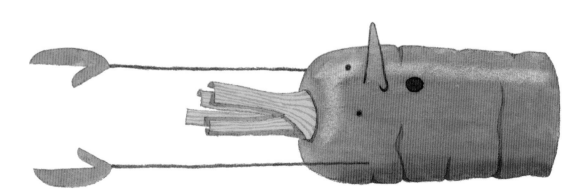

Iron deficiency and anemia can cause difficult behavior and poor concentration in toddlers.

If you are bringing your child up on a vegetarian diet or if he simply dislikes eating meat, make sure that you include nutrient-dense foods like cheese and eggs in his diet. Avoid giving too many high-fiber foods like whole-grain cereals and pulses, as tummies fill up quickly and your child may not get enough energy and protein to grow. Provided your toddler is eating a good variety of food types, a vegetarian diet can provide all the nutrients he needs. It is very important to include vegetarian sources of iron such as green vegetables, dried beans and legumes, fortified breakfast cereals, and dried fruit every day, and make sure you give foods or drinks containing vitamin C at the same meal as this helps to boost the iron absorption from non-meat sources.

Pasta remains a great favorite with toddlers and you can combine it with other healthy foods such as vegetables and tuna. Individual pieces of pasta like penne or fusilli tend to be easiest for toddlers to eat. (Although, when my son, Nicholas, was 20 months old he invented his own method of eating spaghetti – he held it out in front of him by the two ends and sucked in from the middle! Not the height of good manners perhaps, but certainly very efficient.)

Junk food substitutes
Three-quarters of the salt and saturated fat that children consume comes from processed foods and ready meals. Most children eat twice as much salt as they should. It's much better to make your own healthy "junk food" – try my delicious recipes for Annabel's Tasty Beefburgers or Homemade Fast Food Pizza (see pages 178 and 158).

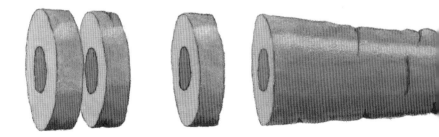

Here are some substitutes for "junk food":

Sugar-coated breakfast cereals	Oatmeal, Cheerios, or muesli
Chicken nuggets	Chicken on the Griddle (page 174) or Bar-B-Q Chicken (page 171)
Fish sticks	Fish Pie (page 164) or Salmon Cakes (page 160)
Canned spaghetti	Pasta with Hidden-Vegetable Tomato Sauce (page 156)
Sausages	Cocktail Meatballs (page 180) or Mini Minute Steaks (page 181)
Chips	Popcorn
Juice drinks or soda	Pure fruit juice

Fruit and desserts

There are many recipes in this chapter for delicious hot and cold desserts that are easy to prepare and can be enjoyed by the whole family. However, there is still nothing more delicious or better for you than fresh ripe fruit, so make sure your child has plenty of it every day. None of the vitamins or nutrients are destroyed through cooking, and fruit makes great finger food for your toddler.

Fruits are packed with powerful antioxidants and natural compounds called phytochemicals, which help boost immunity and protect the body from heart disease and cancer. The incidence of cancer is increasing. Approximately one-third of cancer cases are related to what we eat, and researchers estimate that a diet filled with fruit and vegetables instead of fats and processed foods, along with exercise, could reduce the incidence of cancer by at least 30 percent.

Whole fruit in a fruit bowl isn't that appealing to a hungry child, but if you have a selection of fresh fruit cut up and placed on a low shelf in the fridge, or bite-sized fruit on a skewer, this will help stop your child from snacking on chips or cookies.

Dried fruits, especially apricots, are very nutritious as the drying process concentrates the nutrients. However, take care to cut dried fruits into very small pieces to avoid choking, and don't give dried fruit too often in between meals, as it sticks to the teeth and even natural sugars cause tooth decay.

Kiwi fruit and citrus and berry fruits are rich in vitamin C, which helps to boost iron absorption, so try to make sure you include these in your child's diet. You can add fresh or dried fruits to breakfast cereals. It's also worth buying a juicer so you can make your own fresh-fruit smoothies. Pure fruit juice and smoothies are also good, but be wary of fruit juice drinks as they often contain as little as 10 percent juice, so always read the label. Juices are a great source of vitamins but remember that only by eating the whole fruit will your child be getting fiber.

As different fruits provide different nutrients, include as much variety as possible in your child's diet. Try introducing him to some more exotic fruits. One kiwi fruit contains more than the daily adult requirement of vitamin C and makes a good snack when cut in half, placed in an egg cup, and eaten with a teaspoon. You could also make a tropical fruit salad with mango, melon balls, pineapple, and a sauce made with fresh orange juice and passion fruit or tropical fruit juice.

You can make delicious and healthy ice pops from puréed fresh fruits, yogurt, fruit juices, or smoothies. Ice-pop molds are cheap to buy, and one food that almost no child can resist is an ice pop, so this is a good way to encourage children to eat more fruit.

Ice creams in all colors, shapes, and sizes are sold all over the world. However, the quality of some products is put to shame by the genuine, homemade experience. If you do buy ice creams, choose those that are made from natural ingredients only. If you want to try your hand at making your own, it really is worth investing in an ice-cream-making machine, which churns the mixture as it freezes. Believe me, you will put it to good use over the years and your children will be very popular with their friends when they come round for tea.

Quantities

In this chapter, I have given quantities in adult portions. Every child is different and you must gauge the portion size on your toddler's appetite. He can eat anything from a quarter of an adult portion to a whole portion if he is exceptionally hungry or greedy!

Food additives, particularly artificial colorings, have been blamed for causing hyperactivity in children and are linked with problems such as ADHD. To cut down on additives, try to make the majority of your family's food yourself. You may well see a big change in your child's behavior.

Overweight children

In the US, 15 percent of children and teenagers are overweight and a further 15 percent are at risk of becoming overweight. If your child is overweight, then you should discuss with your pediatrician the best ways of decreasing his calorie intake. Adopt a healthier eating plan rather than cutting down on the amount of food offered. No child should ever go hungry. Cut out sugary, fatty, and processed foods and give more fresh fruit and vegetables. Give high-fiber and whole-grain cereals like oatmeal or raisin bran. Give baked potatoes instead of fries, griddled or broiled skewers, broiled or roast chicken instead of chicken nuggets, and fish without bread crumbs. Reduced-fat milk can be introduced from two years.

Vegetables

Vegetarian Nasi Goreng ☺ ☹

Toddlers love rice. If you don't want a vegetarian version, you can stir in 6 oz cooked shrimp or 1 cup diced cooked chicken with the rice.

MAKES 4–6 ADULT PORTIONS
1 cup long-grain rice (basmati or jasmine)
2 tablespoons vegetable or canola oil
2 eggs
2 tablespoons soy sauce, plus 1 teaspoon to serve
2 shallots, thinly sliced
1 fat garlic clove, crushed
1 tablespoon dark brown sugar
1 medium carrot, peeled and diced or ½ cup baby corn
¼ red bell pepper, diced
¾ cup frozen peas

Cook the rice following the package instructions. Drain, rinse with cold water, and set aside to drain.

Heat 1 tablespoon of the oil in a wok. Beat the eggs with 1 teaspoon of the soy sauce and 1 tablespoon water. Add to the wok and cook to make a large omelet. Break up with a spoon or spatula and transfer to a plate.

Heat the remaining oil and stir-fry the shallots for 2–3 minutes, until starting to brown. Stir in the garlic and cook for 1 minute, then stir in the sugar and cook for 1–2 minutes, stirring until the sugar has melted. Add the carrot (or corn) and bell pepper and cook for 3–4 minutes until the carrot/corn is starting to soften, then add the rice and peas and stir-fry for 3–4 minutes until the rice is hot and the peas have thawed. Stir in the omelet pieces and serve with extra soy sauce, if needed.

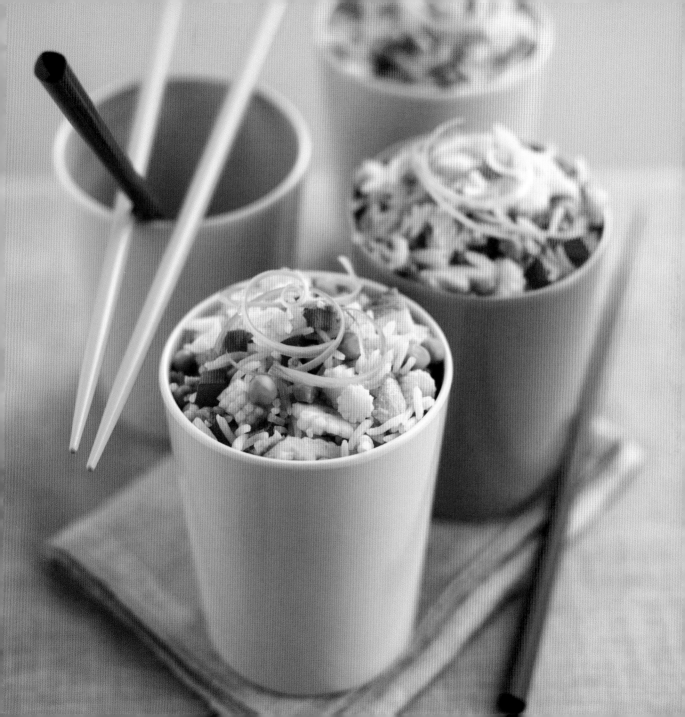

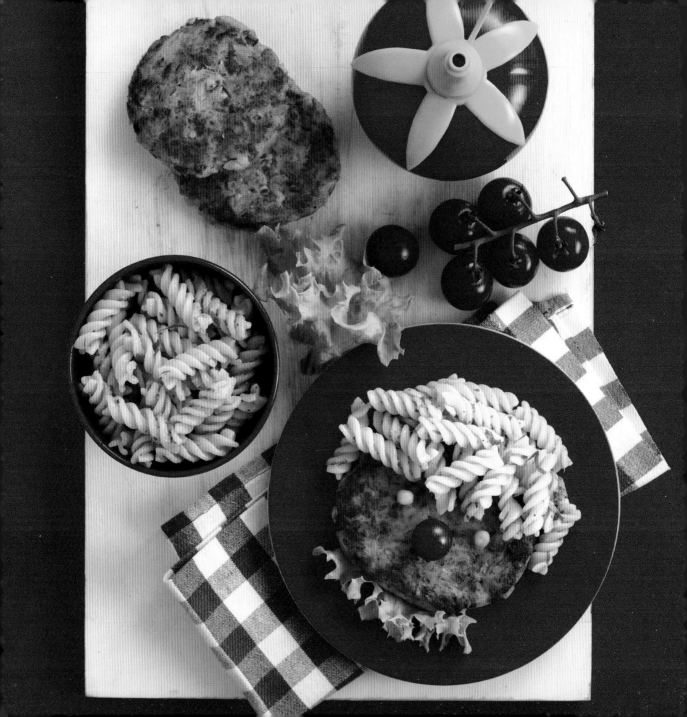

Annabel's Vegetable Burgers ❄ ☺ ☹

These are very popular in my house and even confirmed veggie-haters seem to like them. If you want to freeze these burgers, it's best to cook them first, then put them on a tray lined with plastic wrap. When they are frozen, wrap them in plastic wrap individually. You can then remove them from the freezer as you need them.

MAKES 8 BURGERS

12 oz medium potatoes (such as Yukon gold), skins left on
1½ tablespoons olive oil
¾ cup finely chopped red onion
¾ cup finely chopped leek (white and pale green parts)
1½ cups peeled and grated carrot
1¼ cups diced cremini mushrooms
1 garlic clove, crushed
1 teaspoon fresh thyme leaves
1 tablespoon soy sauce
½ cup grated Gruyère cheese
1¼ cups fresh bread crumbs
2 teaspoons honey
1 small egg yolk
salt and freshly ground black pepper
all-purpose flour for dusting
vegetable or canola oil for frying

Prick the potatoes and cook them in the microwave on High for about 10 minutes, until soft. Alternatively, boil them in a pan of water for 30 minutes. Set aside to cool. Meanwhile, heat the olive oil in a large frying pan and sauté the onion, leek, carrot, mushrooms, garlic, and thyme for 10 minutes, stirring occasionally, until the vegetables are soft. Make sure the mixture is quite dry. Set aside to become cold.

Peel the potatoes and lightly mash with a fork. Add the cold vegetables and the soy sauce, cheese, crumbs, honey, and egg yolk. Mix together and season well. Shape into 8 burgers and chill in the fridge for 30 minutes. Lightly flour the burgers on both sides, then fry in a little oil for 3–4 minutes on each side until golden and cooked through.

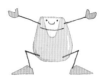

Baked Risotto ☺ ☹

This recipe isn't at all time-consuming to make, as it looks after itself.

MAKES 4 SMALL PORTIONS
2 tablespoons butter
1 small onion, finely chopped
1 garlic clove, crushed
½ teaspoon fresh thyme leaves
¾ cup Arborio rice
1 tablespoon white wine vinegar
scant 2 cups hot chicken or vegetable broth (see pages 76 and 38)
1¼ cups frozen peas
½ cup grated Parmesan cheese
salt and freshly ground black pepper
½ teaspoon lemon juice

Preheat the oven to 400°F. Melt the butter in a wok or large frying pan and sauté the onion for 4–5 minutes, until soft. Add the garlic, thyme, and rice and cook, stirring, for 2 minutes. Add the vinegar and cook until it has evaporated, then stir in the broth and transfer everything to a baking dish (about 6-cup/1½-quart capacity). Cover the dish with aluminum foil and bake for 20–25 minutes, until the broth has been absorbed and the rice is tender. Remove from the oven and stir in the peas and Parmesan, then re-cover and let stand for 2–3 minutes until the peas have warmed through. (You can return the dish to the oven if the kitchen is cold.) Season to taste with salt and pepper and stir in the lemon juice before serving.

Risotto is nice on its own, but you can serve it as a side dish with roast chicken, or try stirring in 4 oz cooked salad-size shrimp, flaked poached salmon, or diced cooked chicken.

My Favorite Spanish Omelet ☺ ☹

This is good served cold and cut into wedges the next day. I give suggestions below for additions to the basic omelet.

MAKES 4 ADULT PORTIONS

3 tablespoons olive oil

1⅓ cups potato (about 6 oz unprepared), peeled and diced

1 onion, peeled and finely chopped

½ small red bell pepper, seeded and chopped

½ cup frozen peas

4 eggs

2 tablespoons Parmesan cheese, grated

salt and pepper

SUGGESTED VARIATIONS

2 tablespoons Gruyère instead of Parmesan cheese

1 large tomato, chopped

or

⅔ cup mushrooms, sliced

1 tablespoon fresh chives, snipped

or

⅔ cup cooked ham or bacon, cubed

½ cup canned corn, drained, instead of peas

Heat the oil in a non-stick 7-inch skillet. Fry the potato and onion for 5 minutes, then add the bell pepper and continue to cook for 5 minutes. Add the peas and cook for a further 5 minutes. Beat the eggs together with 1 tablespoon of water and the Parmesan, and season with salt and pepper. Pour this mixture over the vegetables and cook for 5 minutes or until the omelet is almost set. To finish, brown the top under a preheated broiler for about 3 minutes or until golden. (You can wrap the handle of the skillet with aluminum foil to prevent it burning, if necessary.) Cut into wedges and serve with salad.

Annabel's Hidden-Vegetable Tomato Sauce ❄ ☺ ☹

This is the perfect recipe for children who won't eat their vegetables, as all the vegetables are blended into the tomato sauce so they can't be identified or picked out. This tasty sauce can be used as a topping for pizzas or as a sauce for chicken and rice.

MAKES 4 ADULT PORTIONS
2 tablespoons light olive oil
1 garlic clove, crushed
1 medium onion, peeled and finely chopped
1 cup carrot, peeled and grated
½ cup zucchini, grated
⅔ cup cremini mushrooms, sliced
1 teaspoon balsamic vinegar
1 x 14-oz can tomato sauce with no added salt
1 teaspoon soft brown sugar
1 vegetable bouillon cube dissolved in 1⅔ cups boiling water
a handful fresh basil leaves, torn
salt and freshly ground black pepper

Heat the oil in a saucepan, add the crushed garlic, and sauté for a few seconds, then add the onion and sauté for a further 2 minutes. Add the carrot, zucchini, and mushrooms and sauté for 4 minutes, stirring occasionally. Add the balsamic vinegar and cook for 1 minute. Stir in the tomato sauce and sugar, cover, and simmer for 8 minutes. Add the vegetable broth (from the bouillon cube) and cook for 2 minutes, stirring continuously. Add the basil and season to taste. Transfer to a blender and blitz until smooth.

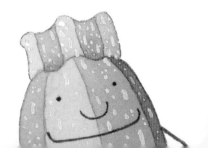

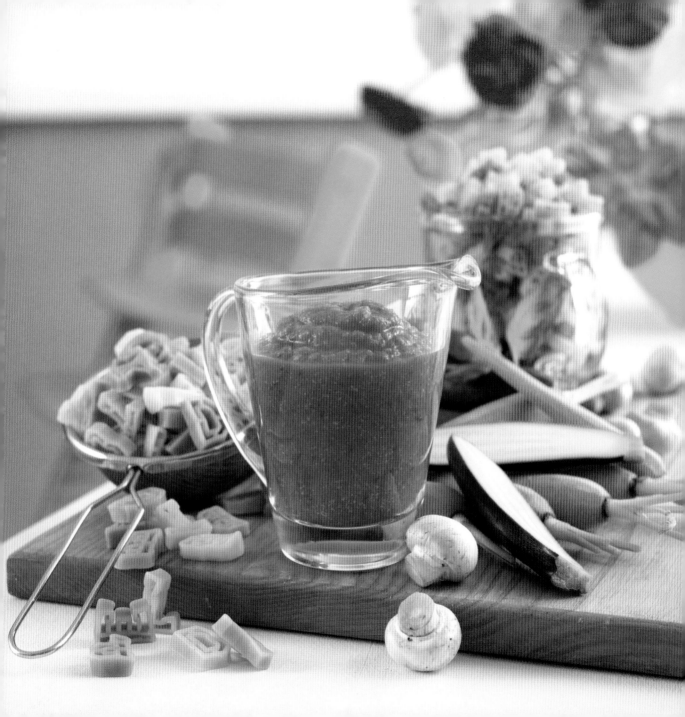

Homemade Fast-Food Pizza ☺ ☹

These delicious easy-to-make pizzas are always popular. If you prefer, you can use crumpets, halved small baguettes, or split pitta breads grilled for a minute or two as the base of the pizzas.

MAKES 2 INDIVIDUAL PIZZAS
1 English muffin, split in half
1 tablespoon good-quality tomato sauce
1 teaspoon red pesto (or regular pesto if red pesto isn't available)
1 tablespoon olive oil
½ small red onion, peeled and chopped
2 small mushrooms, sliced
½ small zucchini (about 2 oz), thinly sliced
1 slice ham or salami, cut into pieces (optional)
½ cup Cheddar or mozzarella cheese, grated
salt and freshly ground black pepper

Toast the muffin until golden and leave to cool. Preheat the broiler to High. Mix the tomato sauce and pesto and spread over the muffins. Heat the olive oil in a skillet and cook the onion for 2 minutes, then add the mushrooms and zucchini and cook until softened and golden. Season to taste.

Divide the vegetable mixture between the muffin bases and spread over evenly. Sprinkle over the ham or salami (if using) and top with the cheese. Place under the preheated broiler and cook for about 4 minutes or until golden and bubbling.

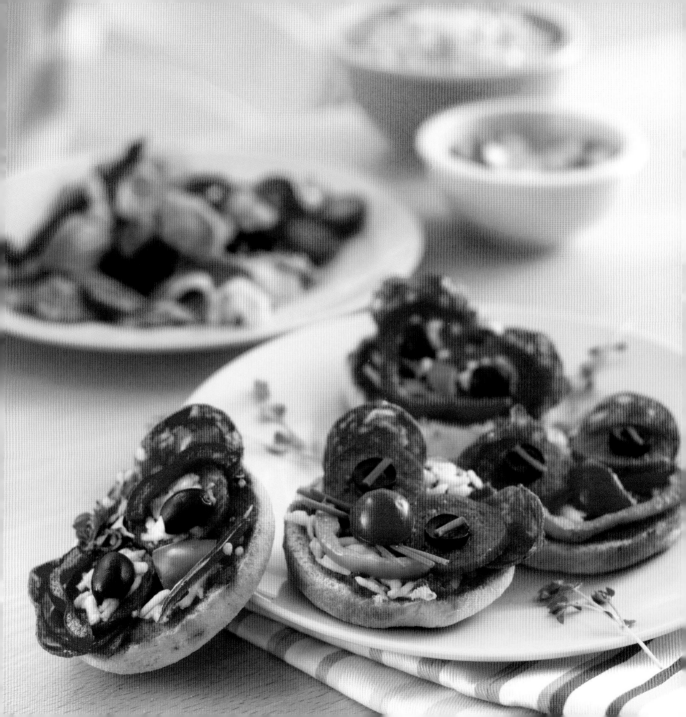

Fish

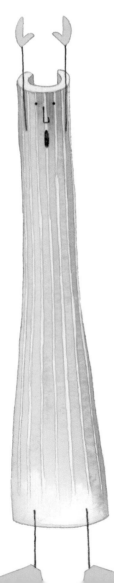

My Favorite Salmon Cakes ❄ ☺ ☹

Salmon is a good source of omega-3 fatty acids, which are great brain boosters. Doctors recommend including at least two oil-rich fish dishes a week to keep the heart in good shape. This super simple, tasty recipe for salmon cakes is very popular with kids and a great meal for all the family.

MAKES 8 CAKES
9 oz potatoes (such as Yukon gold), skins left on
2 tablespoons mayonnaise
1½ tablespoons Thai sweet chili sauce
1 teaspoon lemon juice
2 fat scallions, thinly sliced
⅓ cup grated Cheddar cheese
2 tablespoons ketchup
8 oz salmon fillet, skinned and cut into small cubes
1 cup fresh white bread crumbs
salt and freshly ground black pepper
1 heaping cup dried unseasoned bread crumbs for coating
vegetable or canola oil for frying

DIP
3 tablespoons mayonnaise
2 tablespoons Thai sweet chili sauce

Put the potatoes in a saucepan of cold water. Bring to a boil, then simmer for 20–25 minutes, until you can insert a knife easily. Drain and set aside until cool enough to handle, then peel and spoon the flesh into a bowl. Mix with the mayonnaise, sweet chili sauce, lemon juice, scallions, Cheddar, and ketchup and roughly mash. Mix in the salmon and fresh bread crumbs and season to taste. Form the mixture into 8 cakes. Coat in the dried bread crumbs. Heat some oil in a frying pan and sauté for about 5 minutes until golden, turning halfway through.

   To make the dip, mix the mayonnaise and sweet chili sauce together. Alternatively, serve with a little ketchup.

Nursery Fish Pie ❄ ☺ ☹

MAKES 6 ADULT PORTIONS
³/₄ lb fillet of cod, skinned, or 6 oz fillets each of cod and salmon
1¹/₂ cups milk
1 bay leaf, preferably Turkish
4 peppercorns
a sprig of fresh parsley
salt and pepper
2 tablespoons butter
2 tablespoons all-purpose flour
¹/₃ cup Cheddar cheese, grated
2 tablespoons fresh chives, snipped
¹/₂ tablespoon dill, chopped (optional)
2 teaspoons lemon juice
1 hard-boiled egg, chopped
²/₃ cup frozen peas, cooked following box instructions

TOPPING
1¹/₂ lb white potatoes (such as Yukon), peeled and cut into large pieces
3 tablespoons butter
2 tablespoons milk

Put the fish in a saucepan with the milk, bay leaf, peppercorns, parsley, and seasoning. Bring to a boil and then simmer, uncovered, for about 5 minutes or until the fish is cooked. Cook the potatoes for the topping in boiling, lightly salted water until soft. Strain, then mash together with 2 tablespoons of the butter and the milk.

Lift out the fish, reserving the cooking liquid. Melt the butter in a saucepan and stir in the flour. Cook gently for 1 minute, then whisk in the fish liquid gradually and bring to a boil. Simmer for 2–3 minutes until smooth, stirring continuously. Take off the heat and stir in the grated cheese until melted. Break the fish into chunks and fold in together with the chives, dill (if using), lemon juice, boiled egg, peas, and seasoning. Place the fish in an ovenproof dish (a 7-inch-diameter and 3-inch-deep round dish is perfect) and top with the mashed potato. Bake in the oven preheated to 350°F for 15–20 minutes. Dot with the remaining butter and broil for about 2 minutes until brown and crispy.

Grandma's Tasty Fish Pie ❄ ☺ ☹

This is one of my mother's recipes and is a great favorite with all the family. There is never any left the next day.

MAKES 6 ADULT PORTIONS
1 lb cod fillets, skinned
seasoned all-purpose flour
1 egg, lightly beaten
scant 2 cups fine dried bread crumbs
vegetable oil, for frying
1 onion, peeled and finely chopped
1½ tablespoons olive oil
½ green bell pepper, cored, seeded, and chopped
1 red bell pepper, cored, seeded, and chopped
1 x 14-oz can diced tomatoes
2 tablespoons tomato paste
1 teaspoon balsamic vinegar
½ teaspoon brown sugar
salt and freshly ground black pepper

CHEESE SAUCE
2 tablespoons butter
3 tablespoons all-purpose flour
1¼ cups milk
¾ cup grated Cheddar cheese
½ cup grated Parmesan cheese
¼ teaspoon English mustard (optional)

Preheat the oven to 350°F. Cut the cod fillets into about 12 pieces, dip in seasoned flour, then into the lightly beaten egg, and finally coat in bread crumbs. Sauté in the vegetable oil until golden on both sides. Drain on paper towels.

Sauté the onion in the olive oil for 3–4 minutes. Add the bell peppers and cook for 8 minutes. Drain half of the juice from the tomatoes, then add the tomatoes and the remaining juice to the peppers with the tomato paste, balsamic vinegar, and sugar. Season to taste and cook for about 5 minutes.

Mix the cooked fish with the tomato sauce and transfer to a fairly shallow ovenproof dish.

Make a cheese sauce with the butter, flour, and milk, stirring over a low heat until smooth and thick (see page 67). Remove from the heat and stir in two-thirds of the Cheddar and Parmesan and the mustard, if using.

Pour the cheese sauce over the fish fillets. Sprinkle with the remaining grated cheese and bake in the preheated oven for about 20 minutes. Brown under a hot broiler.

Fish in Creamy Mushroom Sauce ❄ ☺ ☹

For older children, cook 8 cups (½ lb) fresh baby spinach, lay each whole fillet on a bed of the spinach, and pour on the sauce.

MAKES 4 ADULT PORTIONS
1 small onion, peeled and finely chopped
3 tablespoons butter
3 cups small mushrooms, washed and finely chopped
2 tablespoons lemon juice
2 tablespoons chopped fresh parsley
2 tablespoons all-purpose flour
1¼ cups milk
2 flounders, filleted

Fry the onion in half the butter until transparent. Add the mushrooms, lemon juice, and parsley and cook for 2 minutes. Add the flour and cook for 2 minutes, stirring continuously. Add the milk gradually and cook, stirring continuously, until the sauce is thick and smooth.

Fry the flounder fillets in the rest of the butter for 2–3 minutes on each side. Cut or flake the fish into small pieces and mix with the mushroom sauce. Alternatively, cover the uncooked fish with the mushroom sauce and bake in the oven preheated to 350°F for about 15 minutes or until the fish just flakes.

Mommy's Favorite Fish Pie ❄ ☺ ☹

If you want your child to grow up liking fish, then you should try this delicious fish pie. It's good to freeze individual portions in ramekin dishes for days when you don't want to cook.

MAKES 4 MINI FISH PIES
1¼ lb white potatoes (such as Yukon), peeled and cut into large pieces
¼ cup milk
¾ stick butter
1 small onion, finely chopped
2 tomatoes, skinned, seeded, and chopped
1½ tablespoons all-purpose flour
scant 1 cup milk
½ lb cod fillets, skinned, and cut into fairly large cubes
½ lb salmon fillets, skinned, and cut into fairly large cubes
1 tablespoon parsley, chopped
1 bay leaf
½ cup Cheddar cheese, grated
1 egg, lightly beaten
a little salt and freshly ground black pepper (for children over one)

Cook the potatoes in a pan of lightly salted water until tender (about 15 minutes), then strain and mash together with the ¼ cup of milk and half of the butter and season to taste.

Melt the remaining butter in a heavy-based saucepan and sauté the onion for 3 minutes. Add the chopped tomatoes and sauté for 2–3 minutes. Stir in the flour and cook for 1 minute. Add the milk, bring to the boil, and cook for 1 minute. Stir in the cod, salmon, parsley, and bay leaf and simmer for 3–4 minutes. Remove the bay leaf, stir in the grated Cheddar until melted, and season to taste.

Preheat the oven to 350°F. Divide the fish between 4 ramekin dishes (about 4 inches in diameter) and top with the mashed potato. Brush the potato with lightly beaten egg and bake in the oven for 15–20 minutes. You can brown them under a preheated broiler for a few minutes at the end if you wish.

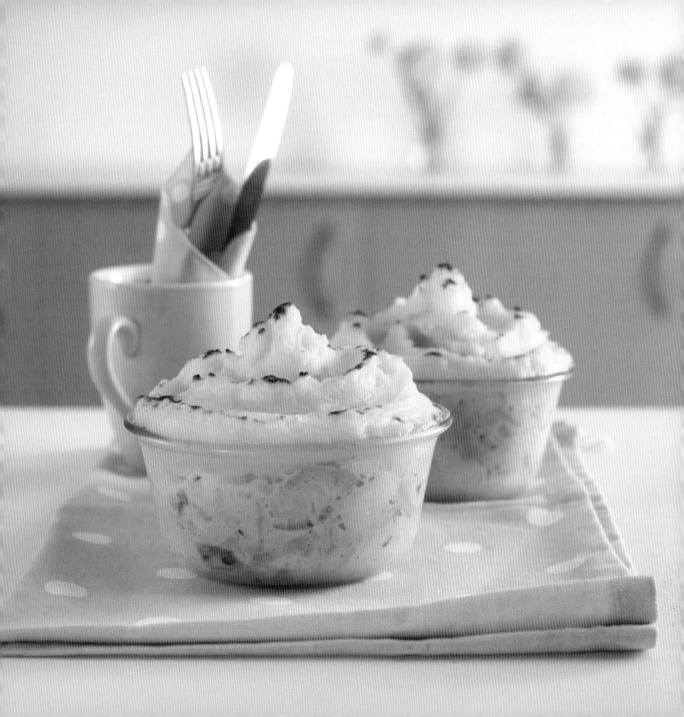

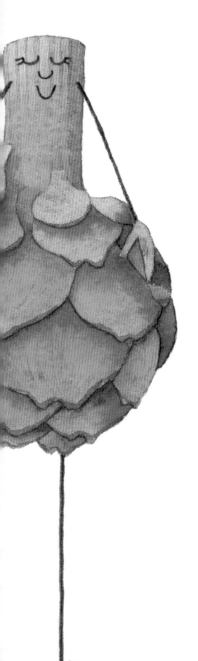

Mild Korma Curry with Shrimp ❄ ☺ ☹

Shrimp are a good source of iron, zinc, and the trace mineral selenium, which is a useful antioxidant. Children often like their mild and slightly sweet flavor.

MAKES 3 PORTIONS
2 tablespoons olive oil
1 small onion, peeled and finely chopped
1 teaspoon grated gingerroot
1 tablespoon korma curry paste (such as Patak's)
1 teaspoon garam masala
half of a 14-oz can diced tomatoes
1 cup coconut milk
½ teaspoon lemon juice
1 teaspoon mango chutney
8 oz uncooked extra-large shrimp, peeled
salt and freshly ground black pepper

Heat the oil in a saucepan. Add the onion and sauté for 3 minutes. Add the ginger, curry paste, and garam masala and fry for 2 minutes. Add the tomatoes, coconut milk, lemon juice, and mango chutney. Bring to a boil, then simmer, uncovered, for 8–10 minutes, stirring until it has reduced and is orangey-red in color. Add the shrimp and simmer for another 5 minutes, until the shrimp have turned pink and are cooked through. Season to taste.

Toasted Tuna Muffins ❄ ☺ ☹

A can of tuna in the larder is a good standby and tuna is rich in protein, vitamin D, and vitamin B12. These toasted English muffins are quick and easy to make for a tasty and healthy meal.

MAKES 1–2 PORTIONS
1 x 4-oz can tuna in oil, drained
1 tablespoon sour cream or mayonnaise
1 tablespoon tomato ketchup
1 scallion, finely chopped
2 tablespoons canned corn, drained
1 English muffin
¼ cup Cheddar cheese, grated

Flake the tuna into a bowl and stir in the sour cream or mayonnaise, tomato ketchup, scallion, and corn. Preheat the broiler, divide the muffin into two halves, and toast. Divide the tuna mixture between the two halves. Cover with the grated cheese and place under the broiler for about 2 minutes until golden and bubbling.

Tuna Pita Pockets ☺ ☹

MAKES 2 PITA POCKETS
1 x 4-oz can tuna in oil, drained
½ cup canned corn, drained
1 hard-boiled egg, chopped
1 tablespoon mayonnaise
½ teaspoon white wine vinegar
2 scallions, chopped
1 tomato, skinned, seeded, and chopped
salt and freshly ground black pepper
1 pita bread

Flake the tuna with a fork and mix with the corn, hard-boiled egg, mayonnaise, white wine vinegar, scallions, tomato, and seasoning. Toast the pita bread, cut in half to make two pockets, and divide the mixture between them.

Tuna Pasta Bake ☺ ☹

MAKES 6 PORTIONS
8 oz fusilli pasta, cooked following the package instructions

TUNA AND TOMATO SAUCE
1 small onion, peeled and finely chopped
2 tablespoons butter
1 tablespoon cornstarch
$1\frac{2}{3}$ cups ready-to-eat cream of tomato soup
$\frac{1}{2}$ teaspoon mixed dried herbs
1 tablespoon chopped fresh parsley
2 x 5-oz cans tuna in oil, drained and flaked
freshly ground black pepper

CHEESY MUSHROOM SAUCE
1 small onion, peeled and finely chopped
3 tablespoons butter
$1\frac{1}{2}$ cups sliced cremini mushrooms
2 tablespoons all-purpose flour
$1\frac{1}{4}$ cups whole milk
$\frac{2}{3}$ cup grated Cheddar cheese
salt and freshly ground black pepper

3 tablespoons grated Parmesan cheese

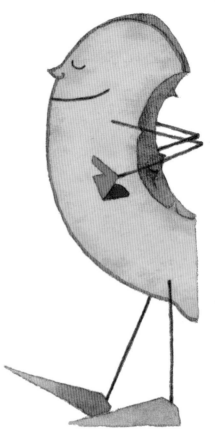

To make the tuna and tomato sauce, fry the onion in the butter until soft. Dissolve the cornstarch in $\frac{1}{2}$ cup water, then add the tomato soup. Add to the onion with the herbs, and stir over low heat for 3 minutes until the sauce thickens slightly. Mix in the tuna and heat through. Season with a little pepper. To make the cheesy mushroom sauce, fry the onion in the butter until soft. Add the mushrooms and cook for 3 minutes. Add the flour and stir for 1 minute. Gradually add the milk, stirring until thickened. Remove from the heat and stir in the Cheddar until melted. Season to taste. Mix the tuna and tomato sauce with the drained pasta and spoon into an ovenproof dish. Cover with the mushroom sauce and sprinkle with the Parmesan. Bake at 350°F for 20 minutes, then broil until lightly golden.

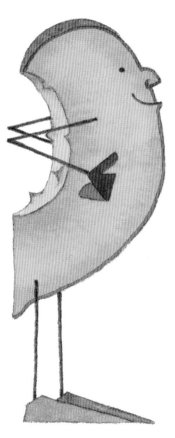

Tuna with Pasta and Tomatoes ☺ ☺

The red onion and oven-roasted tomatoes give this pasta dish a lovely flavor. Oven-roasted tomatoes are available from deli counters, usually packed in olive oil. They are sweeter and not as hard as normal sun-dried tomatoes.

MAKES 4 PORTIONS

½ lb penne
2 tablespoons olive oil
1 medium red onion, peeled and finely sliced
4 ripe plum tomatoes, quartered, seeded, and roughly chopped
1 x 7-oz can tuna in oil, drained
¾ cup oven-roasted tomatoes, chopped
   (or ½ cup sun-dried tomatoes in oil, chopped)
1 teaspoon balsamic vinegar
a handful of fresh basil leaves, torn
salt and freshly ground black pepper

Cook the penne in boiling salted water following the box instructions. Meanwhile, heat the oil in a skillet, add the onion, and cook for about 6 minutes, stirring occasionally until softened. Stir in the fresh tomatoes and cook for 2–3 minutes until beginning to soften. Add the tuna, oven-roasted tomatoes, balsamic vinegar, basil, and seasoning and cook for 1 minute, then stir into the pasta and serve.

Chicken

Thai-style Chicken and Noodles ❄ ☺ ☹

Don't be afraid to try out new tastes on your child – this recipe, flavored with mild curry and coconut sauce, is very popular. Young children often surprise us and like quite sophisticated foods, and it's usually easier to get children to accept new tastes whilst they are young. This would make a good meal for the whole family.

MAKES 4 PORTIONS
MARINADE
1 tablespoon soy sauce
1 tablespoon sake
1/2 teaspoon sugar
1 teaspoon cornstarch

1 1/2 chicken breast fillets, cut into strips
1/4 lb Chinese noodles, such as Chow Mein noodles
1 tablespoon vegetable oil
3 scallions, sliced
1 garlic clove, crushed
1/2 teaspoon red chile, seeded and chopped
1 1/2–2 teaspoons mild curry paste
2/3 cup chicken broth (see page 76)
2/3 cup coconut milk
1 cup broccoli florets
1 1/2 cups beansprouts
3/4 cup frozen peas

Mix together the ingredients for the marinade and marinate the chicken for at least 30 minutes. Cook the noodles following the instructions on the bag, strain, and rinse under cold water. Heat the vegetable oil in a wok or skillet and stir-fry the scallions, garlic, and chile for about 2 minutes. Drain the marinade from the chicken, add the chicken to the wok, and continue to stir-fry for 2 minutes. Add the curry paste, chicken broth, and coconut milk and cook for 5 minutes over a low heat. Add the broccoli and beansprouts and cook for 3–4 minutes. Add the peas and cook for 2 minutes more. Add the noodles to the pan to heat through.

Bar-B-Q Chicken ☺ ☹

A good marinade will transform your grilling, tenderizing the meat, as well as adding a delicious flavor. I use a Weber Grill, which has a cover, enabling me to grill all year round, even in England. Use 2 lb breast of chicken, skinned and on the bone, with these marinades – they also work well with beef or lamb.

MAKES 4–5 ADULT PORTIONS

HOISIN MARINADE

2 tablespoons soy sauce
2 tablespoons hoisin sauce
2 tablespoons rice wine vinegar
1 tablespoon honey
1 tablespoon vegetable oil
½ teaspoon crushed garlic (optional)

TERIYAKI MARINADE

3 tablespoons rice wine vinegar or white wine vinegar
2 tablespoons soy sauce
1 tablespoon honey
½ tablespoon sesame oil
1 teaspoon ginger root, grated (optional)
1 tablespoon scallion, sliced

Mix all the marinade ingredients together. Marinate the chicken for at least 2 hours, then grill, basting and turning occasionally for 15–25 minutes. Dark meat takes longer to cook than white meat. Chicken should be cooked through (an instant-read thermometer should show 165°F when inserted into the thickest part of the chicken) but not overcooked or it will become dry. If you are unsure about cooking meat thoroughly before the surface is charred, cook it in an oven preheated to 400°F for 25–30 minutes and finish it on the grill for a few minutes to give an authentic flavor.

Chicken Satay ☺ ☹

These grilled chicken skewers are fun to eat and very popular with toddlers. Help your child take the meat off the skewers, then remove the skewers – they could become dangerous in the hands of exuberant children.

MAKES 2 ADULT PORTIONS
2 chicken breast fillets
1 small onion, peeled
1 small red bell pepper, seeded

MARINADE
2 tablespoons peanut butter
1 tablespoon chicken broth (see page 76)
1 tablespoon rice vinegar
1 tablespoon honey
1 tablespoon soy sauce
1 teaspoon garlic, crushed (optional)
1 teaspoon sesame seeds, toasted (optional)

Mix together the marinade ingredients. Soak 4 bamboo skewers in water to prevent them getting scorched. Cut the chicken, onion, and pepper into chunks. Leave the chicken in the marinade for at least 2 hours. Thread the chicken, onion, and pepper onto the skewers (or just use chicken). Cook under a preheated broiler for about 5 minutes each side, basting occasionally. Alternatively, cook on a grill or griddle.

Tasty Chicken and Potato Pie ❄ ☺ ☹

This is my version of comfort food – a tasty chicken pie in a delicious white sauce, topped with cheesy mashed potatoes.

MAKES 4 PORTIONS

TOPPING

1¼ pounds potatoes, peeled and cut into chunks
2 tablespoons butter
scant ½ cup whole milk
½ cup grated Cheddar cheese
1 tablespoon grated Parmesan cheese

FILLING

2 tablespoons butter
1 leek, thinly sliced (white and pale green parts)
1 large or 2 small shallots, finely chopped
2 tablespoons all-purpose flour
1½ cups chicken broth (see page 76)
⅓ cup heavy cream
2 cups shredded cooked chicken
⅔ cup frozen peas
1 tablespoon chopped parsley
1 tablespoon lemon juice
salt and freshly ground black pepper

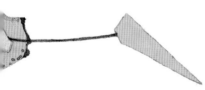

Put the potatoes in cold salted water, bring to a boil, reduce the heat, and simmer for 10–15 minutes, until tender. Drain and mash with the butter, milk, and cheeses.

For the filling, melt the butter in a saucepan and gently cook the leek and shallot for 8–10 minutes, until soft but not colored. Stir in the flour and cook for 1 minute, then gradually stir in the broth to make a smooth sauce (you may find it easiest to do this off the heat). Stir in the cream, then cook, stirring, until the sauce just comes to a boil. Stir in the chicken, peas, and parsley, then remove from the heat, stir in the lemon juice, and season to taste.

Spoon the filling into a 6-cup/1½-quart capacity ovenproof dish and top with the mashed potatoes. Bake in an oven preheated to 400°F for about 20 minutes and then finish off under a preheated broiler for a few minutes until golden. It's a good idea to place the dish on a baking sheet to catch any drips.

Marinated Chicken on the Griddle ☺ ☹

I enjoy cooking chicken, meat, or fish on a griddle, and it's a really healthy way of cooking as it uses very little fat. My three children love this recipe as marinating the chicken gives it a lovely flavor and makes it more tender. Make sure the griddle is really hot before you lay the food on it.

MAKES 2 ADULT PORTIONS
2 chicken breast fillets
1 tablespoon olive oil

MARINADE
1 tablespoon lemon juice
1 tablespoon soy sauce
1 tablespoon honey
1 small garlic clove, peeled and sliced
2 sprigs of fresh rosemary (optional)

Score the chicken breasts 2 or 3 times with a sharp knife. Season with salt and pepper. Mix together all the ingredients for the marinade and marinate the chicken for at least 2 hours. Heat the griddle, brush with oil, then remove the chicken from the marinade and cook for 4–5 minutes on each side or until cooked through. Cut into strips and serve with colorful vegetables such as carrots, broccoli, or peas, and French fries or mashed potato.

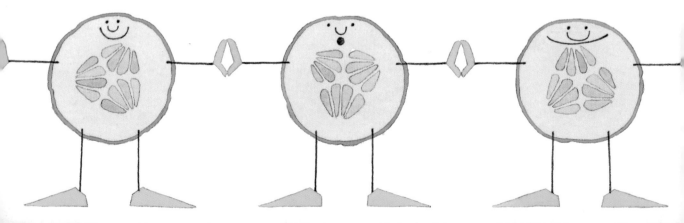

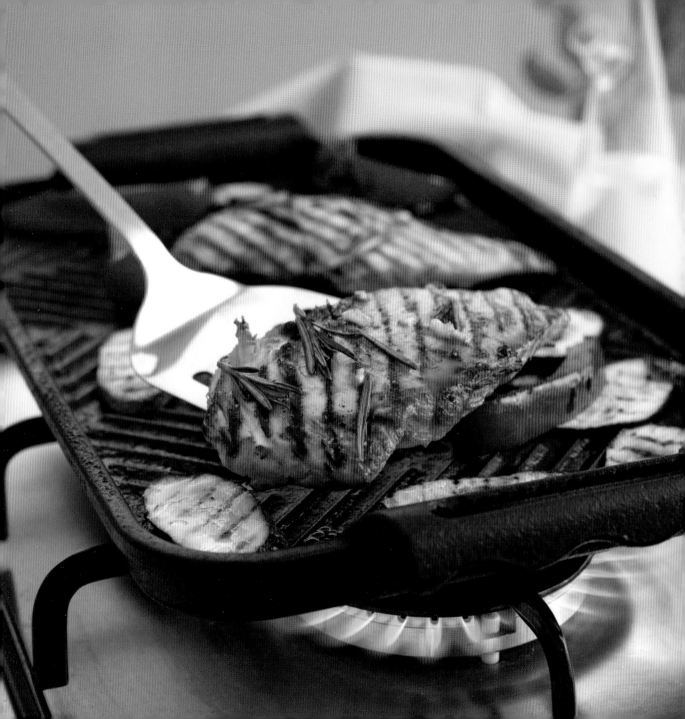

Mulligatawny Chicken ❄ ☺ ☹

This recipe has a tomato base and a fruity curry flavor that children love. It has been a family favorite since I was a child and was invented by my mother. It is best served with rice.

MAKES 4 ADULT PORTIONS
1 tablespoon vegetable oil
1 onion, thinly sliced
1 carrot, peeled and cut into matchsticks
1 garlic clove, crushed
½ red or green chili, seeded and diced (optional)
2 tablespoons korma curry paste (such as Patak's)
1 x 14-oz can diced tomatoes
1 tablespoon tomato paste
1 teaspoon honey
1 apple, peeled, cored, and thinly sliced
½ cup raisins
salt and freshly ground black pepper
8 large bone-in chicken thighs, skin removed

Preheat the oven to 350°F. Heat the oil in a large frying pan. Sauté the onion and carrot for 3–4 minutes, until softened. Add the garlic, chili (if using), and curry paste and cook for 2 minutes. Add the tomatoes, tomato paste, honey, apple, and raisins and season to taste with salt and pepper.

Put the chicken in a casserole or Dutch oven that holds it snugly. Pour on the sauce, then cover tightly with aluminum foil or a lid and bake for 50 minutes to 1 hour, until the chicken is cooked through.

Serve with fluffy white rice. For children, remove the meat from the bones before serving.

Chicken and Butternut Squash Tagine ❄ ☺ ☹

I love the aromatic flavors of a tagine and it's a great way to hide fruit and vegetables from fussy eaters. A tagine is a Moroccan dish, usually made from a mixture of vegetables, chicken or lamb, and dried fruit. My version is simple and quick to prepare and includes the lovely combination of butternut squash, korma curry paste, and dried apricots. I like to use organic dried apricots; they have a much better flavor than ordinary dried apricots, which are treated with sulfur dioxide to preserve their bright-orange color. You can serve this with fluffy white rice or couscous.

MAKES 4 PORTIONS

1 tablespoon olive oil
1 red onion, chopped
1 small carrot, peeled and grated
¼ small butternut squash, peeled and grated
1 garlic clove, crushed
1 tablespoon korma curry paste (such as Patak's)
¼ teaspoon ground cumin
a pinch each of ground cinnamon and ground ginger
a pinch of dried onion flakes (optional)
1 x 14-oz can diced tomatoes
1 tablespoon tomato paste
1 cup vegetable broth
1 teaspoon honey
12 oz skinless, boneless chicken thighs or breasts, cut into bite-sized pieces
8 organic dried apricots, cut into ¼-inch pieces
salt and freshly ground black pepper

Heat the oil in a wok. Sauté the onion, carrot, and squash for 5–6 minutes, until soft. Add the garlic, curry paste, and spices and cook for 2 minutes. Add the tomatoes, tomato paste, broth, and honey. (For fussy eaters, you could blend the sauce at this point to make it smooth.) Bring to a boil and simmer briskly for 10–15 minutes, until thickened. Add the chicken and apricots and reduce the heat slightly, then cook gently for 10 minutes until the chicken is cooked through. Season to taste.

Red meats

Annabel's Tasty Beefburgers ❄ ☺ ☹

The grated apple makes these beefburgers really moist and tasty. Serve in a bun with salad and ketchup, and some oven-baked fries. They are also good cooked on a grill in summer. If you want to freeze burgers, it's best to freeze them uncooked on a tray lined with plastic wrap. Then, when frozen, wrap each one individually in plastic wrap so that you can remove and defrost them as and when you need them.

MAKES 8 BURGERS

½ red bell pepper, cored, seeded, and chopped
1 onion, peeled and finely chopped
1 tablespoon vegetable oil
1 lb lean ground beef or lamb
1 tablespoon fresh parsley, chopped
1 chicken bouillon cube, finely crumbled
1 apple, peeled and grated
1 egg, lightly beaten
½ cup fresh bread crumbs
1 teaspoon Worcestershire sauce, such as Lea and Perrins
salt and freshly ground black pepper
a little all-purpose flour
vegetable oil for brushing a griddle pan or for frying

Fry the bell pepper and half the onion in the vegetable oil for about 5 minutes or until softened. In a mixing bowl, combine the sautéed onion, pepper, and remaining raw onion with all the ingredients except for the flour and extra vegetable oil. With floured hands, form into 8 burgers. Brush a griddle pan with a little oil and, when hot, place 4 burgers on the griddle and cook for about 5 minutes each side or until browned and cooked through. Repeat with the remaining burgers. Alternatively, fry in a little hot oil in a shallow skillet. Serve the burgers on their own or in a toasted hamburger bun with salad and ketchup.

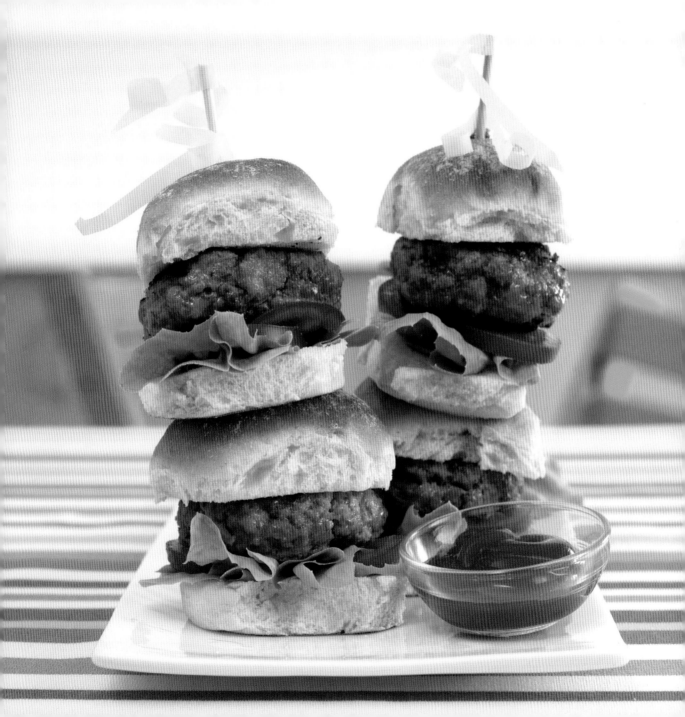

Cocktail Meatballs with Tomato Sauce ❄ ☺ ☹

MAKES 6 PORTIONS

TOMATO SAUCE

1½ tablespoons light olive oil
1 medium onion, peeled and chopped
1 garlic clove, crushed
9 oz fresh ripe tomatoes, skinned, seeded, and chopped
1 x 14-oz can diced tomatoes
1 teaspoon balsamic vinegar
1 teaspoon sugar
salt and freshly ground black pepper
1 tablespoon fresh basil, torn

MEATBALLS

¾ lb lean ground beef
1 medium onion, peeled and finely chopped
1 Granny Smith apple, peeled and grated
1 cup fresh white bread crumbs
1 tablespoon fresh parsley, chopped
1 chicken bouillon cube, finely crumbled and dissolved in 2 tablespoons boiling water
salt and freshly ground black pepper
all-purpose flour for forming meatballs
vegetable oil for frying

To make the tomato sauce, heat the oil in a saucepan, and gently cook the onion and garlic until softened. Stir in the fresh tomatoes and cook for 1 minute. Add the canned tomatoes, vinegar, sugar, and seasoning and cook for 20 minutes over a low heat. Add the basil and then blend in a food processor to make a smooth sauce.

Meanwhile, mix together the ingredients for the meatballs. Using floured hands, form into about 24 balls. Heat the oil in a skillet and sauté the meatballs over a fairly high heat, turning occasionally, until browned, then reduce the heat and continue to cook for about 5 minutes. Pour over the tomato sauce and continue to cook, covered, for 10–15 minutes.

Mini Minute Steaks ☺ ☹

These mini steaks with a full-flavored gravy and sautéed potatoes are absolutely delicious.

MAKES 2 ADULT OR 4 CHILD PORTIONS
2 tablespoons vegetable oil
1 onion, peeled and thinly sliced
1 teaspoon sugar
1 tablespoon water
scant 1 cup beef broth
1 teaspoon cornstarch mixed with
1 tablespoon water
a few drops of Worcestershire sauce, such as Lea and Perrins
1 teaspoon tomato paste
salt and pepper
3/4 lb potatoes, peeled
2 tablespoons butter
4 x 2½ oz minute steaks (tenderloin or sirloin), about ¼ inch thick

To make the gravy, heat 1 tablespoon of the vegetable oil in a skillet. Add the onion and cook for 7–8 minutes until just turning golden brown. Stir in the sugar and water, increase the heat, and cook for about 1 minute until the water has evaporated. Stir in the beef broth, cornstarch mixed with 1 tablespoon water, Worcestershire sauce, and tomato paste. Season with salt and pepper. Cook, stirring, for 2–3 minutes until thickened.

For the sautéed potatoes, cut the potatoes into large chunks, bring to the boil in lightly salted water, and cook for about 8 minutes until they are just tender. Drain and cut into ½ inch-thick slices. Heat the butter in a skillet and sauté the potatoes for 5–6 minutes, turning occasionally until golden brown and crispy.

Heat the remaining oil in a skillet, season the steaks, and fry for 1–2 minutes each side. Serve with the gravy and sautéed potatoes.

Shredded Beef with Broccoli ❄ ☺ ☹

A quick and easy-to-prepare beef stir-fry with a tasty sauce. To toast sesame seeds, stir-fry them in a dry skillet for a couple of minutes until golden, stirring to make sure that they don't burn.

MAKES 4 ADULT PORTIONS
heaping 3/4 cup rice
1 tablespoon sesame oil
1/2 tablespoon canola oil
1 onion, peeled and chopped
1 garlic clove, crushed
1 medium carrot, peeled and cut into matchsticks
1 cup broccoli florets
1/2 lb beef tenderloin, cut into fine strips
1 tablespoon cornstarch
2/3 cup beef broth
2 tablespoons dark brown sugar
1 1/2 tablespoons soy sauce
1 tablespoon toasted sesame seeds (optional)

Cook the rice following the instructions on the bag. Heat the sesame oil and canola oil in a wok or skillet and stir-fry the onion and garlic for 3–4 minutes. Add the carrot and broccoli and stir-fry for 2 minutes. Add the beef strips and stir-fry for 4–5 minutes. Mix the cornstarch with 1 tablespoon of cold water and stir into the beef broth. Stir this into the pan, together with the sugar, soy sauce, and toasted sesame seeds, if using. Bring to a simmer and cook for 2 minutes. Serve with the cooked rice.

Pasta

Spaghetti with Two-Tomato Sauce ❄ ☺ ☹

A really good homemade tomato sauce is always popular – it can be served with any type of pasta and maybe freshly grated Parmesan cheese.

MAKES 4 PORTIONS
3 tablespoons olive oil
1 onion, peeled and chopped
1 garlic clove, peeled and crushed
4 ripe tomatoes, skinned, seeded, and chopped
1 x 14-oz can diced tomatoes
a pinch of sugar
1 bay leaf, preferably Turkish
2 tablespoons fresh basil, chopped
salt and pepper
½ lb spaghetti

Heat the oil in a saucepan and sauté the onion and garlic for 5–6 minutes until softened. Add the fresh and canned tomatoes, sugar, bay leaf, and chopped basil, then season with salt and pepper. Bring to a simmer and cook for 20 minutes. Meanwhile, cook the spaghetti following the box instructions. Strain the pasta and mix with the sauce.

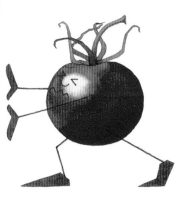

Bow Ties with Cherry Tomatoes and Mozzarella ☺ ☹

A great favorite with my children, this can be eaten either warm or cold.

MAKES 4 PORTIONS
6 oz bow-tie pasta (farfalle)
1 cup halved cherry or grape tomatoes
8 oz mozzarella cheese, cubed
½ heart of romaine lettuce, shredded

DRESSING
2 tablespoons light olive oil
2 teaspoons rice vinegar
¼ teaspoon honey
½ teaspoon prepared basil pesto
1 tablespoon snipped fresh chives (optional)

Cook the pasta following the package instructions. Drain and (when cool, if preferred) mix together with the tomatoes, mozzarella, and lettuce. Whisk together the dressing ingredients and toss with the salad.

Three-Cheese Pasta Sauce ❄ ☺ ☹

This makes a really delicious, creamy cheese sauce for pasta. If you like, you can add a couple of slices of good-quality cooked ham, shredded.

MAKES 4 PORTIONS
2 tablespoons butter
3 tablespoons all-purpose flour
1¼ cups whole milk
½ cup grated Gruyère cheese
heaping ⅓ cup grated Parmesan cheese, plus extra for serving
⅔ cup mascarpone cheese
8 oz penne pasta

To make the sauce, melt the butter, stir in the flour, and cook for 1 minute. Gradually add the milk, then continue to stir for 5 minutes over low heat until the sauce thickens. Remove from the heat, stir in the Gruyère and Parmesan until melted, then stir in the mascarpone.

Cook the pasta following the package instructions and mix with the sauce. Serve with some extra grated Parmesan cheese.

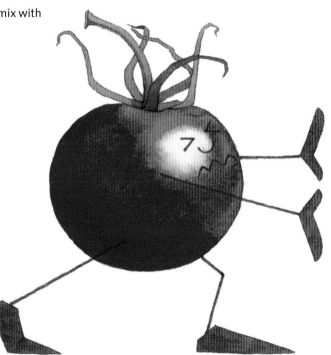

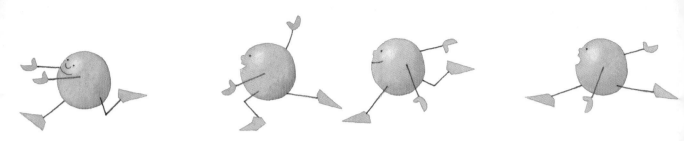

Spaghetti Primavera ❄ ☺ ☹

A simple recipe for spaghetti with spring vegetables in a tasty cheese sauce.
You could also make this with pasta shapes.

MAKES 4 PORTIONS
8 oz spaghetti
1 tablespoon olive oil
1 onion, chopped
1 garlic clove, crushed
1 medium carrot (about 3 oz), cut into matchsticks
1 medium zucchini (about 3 oz), cut into matchsticks
1¼ cups cauliflower florets
²⁄₃ cup light crème fraîche or heavy cream
²⁄₃ cup vegetable broth (see page 38)
½ cup frozen peas
²⁄₃ cup grated Parmesan cheese

Cook the spaghetti following the package instructions. At the same time, heat the
oil in a heavy-bottomed saucepan and sauté the onion and garlic for 1 minute.
Add the carrot and zucchini matchsticks and sauté, stirring occasionally, for
2–3 minutes. Meanwhile, blanch the cauliflower in lightly salted boiling water
for 5 minutes or steam until tender. Add the crème fraîche or cream, vegetable
broth, and peas to the carrots and zucchini and stir in. Cook for 2–3 minutes
before stirring in the Parmesan. Drain the spaghetti and toss with the sauce.

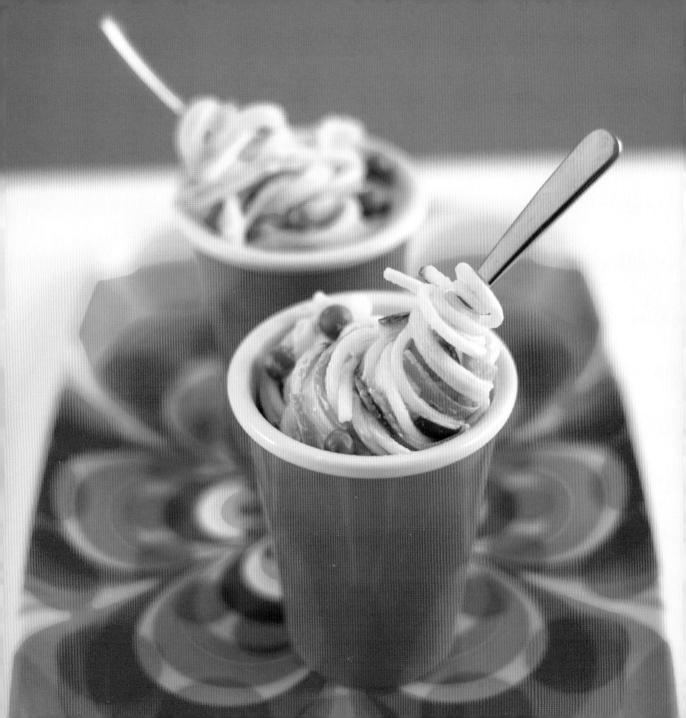

Fruit

Apple Crumble ❄ ☺ ☹

A really good crumble bursting with fruit is comfort food at its very best, and it's quick and easy to prepare. Below is my favorite recipe for apple crumble. If you like, you can stir in 5 oz fresh blackberries once the apples are cooked and add another half tablespoon of sugar. Another good combination is 14 oz rhubarb, thinly sliced and mixed with 4 oz strawberries and 1/4 cup sugar. This is good served hot with vanilla ice cream.

MAKES 6 PORTIONS
1¾ lb apples, peeled, cored, and sliced
juice of 1 orange
2 tablespoons butter
2 tablespoons sugar

CRUMBLE TOPPING
scant 1 cup all-purpose flour
a generous pinch of salt
5 tablespoons cold butter, cut into pieces
⅓ cup turbinado sugar
⅓ cup almond meal (ground almonds)

Preheat the oven to 350°F. Put the apples into a bowl and pour on the orange juice . Melt the butter in a large pan, drain the apples, reserving the orange juice, and sauté the apples with the sugar for about 8 minutes, then stir in 2 tablespoons of the reserved orange juice.

Meanwhile, to prepare the topping, whiz the flour, salt, butter, and sugar in a food processor for a few seconds until the mixture resembles bread crumbs, then pulse in the almond meal. Alternatively, mix together the flour, salt, and sugar, then rub in the butter using your fingers and stir in the almond meal.

Spoon the cooked apples into an 8-inch round glass ovenproof dish and cover with the crumble topping. Alternatively, you could make 4–6 individual portions in ramekins. Bake in the oven for about 30 minutes.

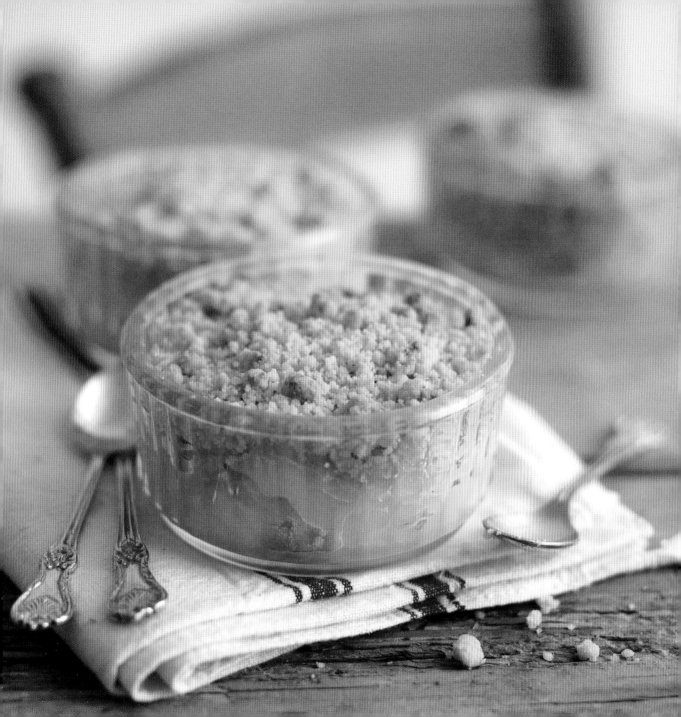

Mini Cheesecakes ❄ ☺ ☹

Really simple and quick to prepare, these individual mini-cheesecakes are made in muffin cases and don't need any baking. Everyone in my family thinks they are yummy. Great for a tea party or birthday celebration. They are also fun for children to make themselves. If you don't want to make these in paper cases you could also make them in small glass ramekins. Lemon curd can be found in the jams and jellies aisle in larger supermarkets and grocery stores.

MAKES 6 MINI CHEESECAKES
½ stick butter
1 cup graham cracker crumbs
8 oz container mascarpone cheese
⅓ cup lemon curd
1 tablespoon lemon juice
½ cup heavy cream
3 teaspoons lemon curd (optional)

Line a muffin pan with 6 large paper muffin cups. Melt the butter and stir in the crumbs. Divide the crumbs between the muffin cups and use clean fingers to press firmly into the base. Chill in the refrigerator whilst you prepare the filling.

Beat together the mascarpone cheese, lemon curd, and lemon juice in an electric mixer. Whip the cream until it just holds its shape (soft peaks). Fold the cream into the cheese mixture. Spoon the filling into the paper cups. If you like, you can top each one with half a teaspoon of lemon curd and swirl this with a toothpick to make a pattern.

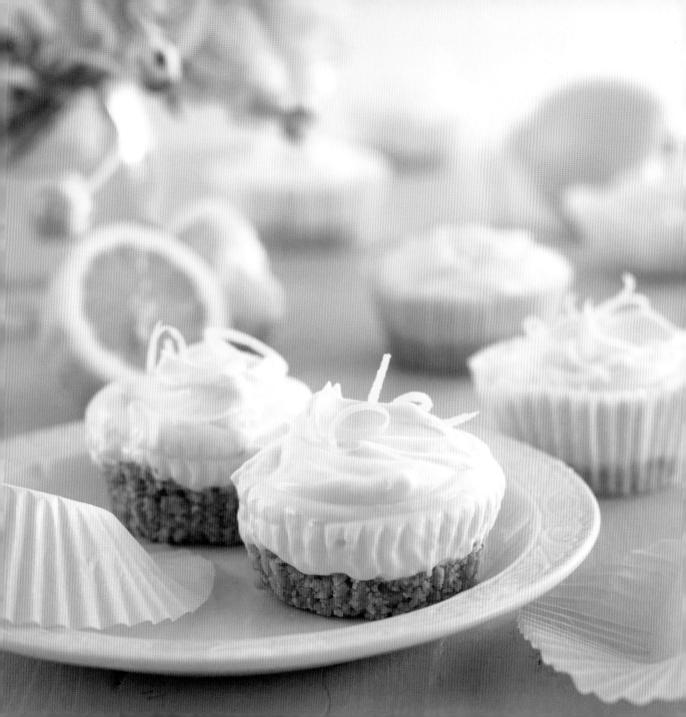

Mini Bread and Butter Puddings ☺ ☹

This is the perfect dessert for when the cupboard is pretty bare. I like to make individual portions in ramekins.

MAKES 4 RAMEKINS
4 small slices white bread
2 tablespoons butter, softened
1 heaping tablespoon apricot jam
½ cup golden raisins
1 teaspoon vanilla extract
1 egg
⅔ cup heavy cream
scant ½ cup whole milk
¼ cup sugar
2 tablespoons turbinado sugar

Spread one side of the bread slices with butter, then top with the jam. Cut off the crusts, then slice each piece of bread into 4 triangles. Arrange the triangles in 4 ramekins (diameter about 4 inches). Scatter the raisins on top. Mix together the vanilla extract, egg, cream, milk, and sugar, then pour into the ramekins. Sprinkle with the turbinado sugar. Let stand for 20 minutes. Bake in a preheated 350°F oven for 20 minutes until puffy and lightly golden brown. Serve immediately.

Ice Pops

Make up your own flavors. Experiment with different combinations like puréed and strained fresh berries sweetened with a little confectioner's sugar and mixed with cranberry or blackcurrant juice. You can also mix in some yogurt such as mini-probiotic drinking yogurts. Try blending a can of lychees with a little lemon or lime juice and strain for a refreshing ice pop.

Strawberry Sorbet Ice Pops ❄ ☺ ☹

If there is one food that no child can resist, it's an ice pop. Most store-bought ice pops are full of artificial flavoring and coloring so it's much better to make your own from fresh fruit. Strawberries contain higher levels of vitamin C than any other berries. Two-tone ice pops are fun. Half-fill the molds with the strawberry sorbet, freeze for a couple of hours, and then pour over an orange-colored juice like apple and mango or tropical fruit juice.

MAKES ABOUT 1 CUP OR 4 SMALL POPS
2 tablespoons superfine sugar
3 tablespoons water
½ lb strawberries, hulled and cut in half
juice of 1 medium orange (about 3 tablespoons)

Put the sugar and water into a saucepan and boil until syrupy (about 3 minutes). Allow to cool. Purée the strawberries with an electric hand (immersion) blender and combine with the cooled syrup and orange juice, then pour this mixture into ice-pop molds. Freeze until solid.

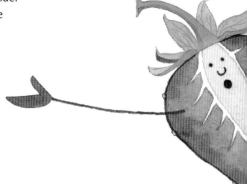

Lychee and Lime Ice Pops ❄ ☺ ☹

MAKES 1 CUP OR 3 SMALL ICE POPS
1 x 20-oz can lychees in syrup, drained
¼ cup syrup from the can
2 tablespoons confectioners' sugar
2½ tablespoons lime juice
finely grated zest of a quarter of a lime

Simply blend everything together and freeze overnight in ice pop molds.

Grandma's Lokshen Pudding ☺ ☹

Lokshen is vermicelli: very fine egg noodles.

MAKES 4 ADULT PORTIONS
½ lb vermicelli
1 large egg, beaten
2 tablespoons butter, melted
1 cup milk
1 tablespoon vanilla sugar or superfine sugar
½ teaspoon mixed spice
⅔ cup each raisins and golden raisins (chopped for smaller children)
a few sliced almonds (optional)

Cook the vermicelli in boiling water for about 5 minutes. Drain and mix with the remaining ingredients. Place in a greased, shallow baking dish, and bake in an oven preheated to 350°F for about 30 minutes.

Frozen Strawberry Yogurt Ice Cream ☺ ☹

A delicious, easy-to-make, frozen-yogurt ice cream using only natural ingredients. You can also make a peach melba frozen yogurt using fresh raspberries, puréed and strained, and peach yogurt. I like to serve this as a layered sundae or parfait, in a tall glass with fresh berries.

MAKES 6 ADULT PORTIONS
½ cup sugar
1¼ cups water
¾ lb fresh strawberries
1¼ cups strawberry yogurt
⅔ cup heavy cream, whipped
1 egg white, whisked

Put the sugar in a saucepan with the water, bring to a boil, and continue to boil for 5 minutes to make a syrup. Set aside to cool for a few minutes. Purée the strawberries and press through a strainer, then mix with the syrup and stir in the yogurt and whipped cream. Churn for 10 minutes in an ice-cream-making machine, then fold in the whisked egg white and churn for another 10 minutes or until firm.

This can also be made without an ice-cream machine but it will be more time-consuming. Pour the mixture into a freezerproof plastic container and freeze. Remove and whisk when semi-frozen, then return to the freezer. Whisk again after 1 hour, fold in the whisked egg white, freeze again, and whisk twice more during the freezing process.

Note: This recipe contains uncooked egg and should be avoided by those who are pregnant, elderly, very young, or have an impaired immune system.

Baking for toddlers

Egg- and Dairy-Free Chocolate Fudge Cake ☺ ☹

MAKES ABOUT 12 SLICES
1 heaping cup all-purpose flour
½ cup unsweetened cocoa powder
1 teaspoon baking soda
¼ teaspoon salt
1 cup (firmly packed) light brown sugar
¼ cup vegetable oil
1 cup hot water (freshly boiled)
1 teaspoon vanilla extract
1 teaspoon white wine vinegar or cider vinegar

FROSTING
¼ cup water
6 tablespoons dairy-free margarine
3 tablespoons light brown sugar
6 oz bittersweet chocolate, chopped (check that it's dairy-free, as brands vary)
½ teaspoon vanilla extract

Preheat the oven to 350°F. Line a 7 x 11-inch cake pan with parchment paper, including the sides and leaving an overhang at two opposite ends.

Whisk the flour, cocoa, baking soda, and salt together in a bowl. Mix together the sugar, oil, water, vanilla, and vinegar in a small bowl. Stir this into the dry ingredients. Pour the batter into the prepared pan (it is quite liquid) and bake for 20–25 minutes, until risen, firm to the touch, and a cake tester comes out clean. Cool in the pan for 15 minutes, then lift out onto a wire rack and let cool completely. Leave the parchment underneath the cake as it makes it easier to move the cake around.

To make the frosting, put all of the ingredients except for the vanilla in a bowl and microwave for 30 seconds. Stir, then microwave in 15-second bursts, stirring between each burst, until everything has melted together. Whisk to make a glossy frosting, then whisk in the vanilla. Alternatively, put the bowl over (but not in) a saucepan of hot water and leave to melt, whisking regularly, then remove the bowl from the saucepan and add the vanilla. Leave in a cool place for 1–2 hours to thicken.

If the frosting is still very liquid, refrigerate the bowl for 5–10 minutes (do not leave any longer), then whisk well. Spread the frosting onto the cooled cake and decorate. You can put the cake into the refrigerator for 10 minutes to firm up the frosting a little more if you like.

Cut into rectangles. (This can also be made into 12 cupcakes. Line a muffin pan with paper liners and half-fill each liner with batter. Bake for 15–17 minutes, until firm to the touch.)

Carrot and Pineapple Muffins ☺ ☹

These are absolutely delicious, and very healthy too; they never last long in our house!

MAKES ABOUT 13 MUFFINS
scant 1 cup all-purpose flour
1 cup wholewheat flour
1 teaspoon baking powder
3/4 teaspoon baking soda
1 teaspoon ground cinnamon
1 teaspoon ground ginger
1/2 teaspoon salt
3/4 cup vegetable oil
1/3 cup superfine sugar
2 eggs
1 1/4 cups carrot, grated
1 x 8-oz can crushed pineapple, drained
2/3 cup raisins (chopped for smaller children)

Preheat the oven to 350°F. In a large bowl, whisk together the flours, baking powder, baking soda, cinnamon, ginger, and salt. Beat the oil, sugar, and eggs together until well blended. Add the grated carrot, crushed pineapple, and raisins. Gradually add the flour mixture, beating just enough to combine all the ingredients.

Pour the batter into muffin pans lined with paper muffin cups and bake for about 25 minutes or until golden. Cool on a wire rack.

Animal Cupcakes ❄ ☺ ☹

Cupcakes are always popular and children will have fun decorating them to look like animals. For best results, the butter and eggs should be at room temperature. To make chocolate cupcakes, substitute 2 tablespoons unsweetened cocoa powder for 2 tablespoons of the self-rising flour and use chocolate buttercream.

MAKES 10 CUPCAKES

9 tablespoons unsalted butter or margarine, at room temperature
²/₃ cup superfine sugar
½ teaspoon grated lemon zest
2 eggs
1 cup self-rising flour
¼ teaspoon baking powder

BUTTERCREAM

7 tablespoons soft unsalted butter
half of a 1-lb box confectioners' sugar, sifted
1 tablespoon milk
½ teaspoon vanilla extract

GLACÉ ICING

half of a 1-lb box confectioners' sugar, sifted
about 2½ tablespoons warm water
a few drops of food coloring

Preheat the oven to 350°F. Line a muffin pan with 10 paper liners. Put the butter, sugar, lemon zest, eggs, flour, and baking powder into a bowl and beat until smooth. Divide the mixture among the paper liners and bake for about 20 minutes, or until golden and springy. Remove from the oven and leave the muffin pan for a few minutes, then transfer the cakes to a wire rack to cool completely.

While the cupcakes are baking, prepare the icings. To make buttercream, beat the butter until soft. Add half the confectioners' sugar and beat until smooth. Beat in the remaining sugar, the milk, and the vanilla. Divide the buttercream into a few bowls and color with a few drops of food coloring. For chocolate buttercream, use 2 cups confectioners' sugar and 2 tablespoons unsweetened cocoa powder.

To make the glacé icing, mix the confectioners' sugar with enough warm water to make a spreading consistency, then divide into three bowls and stir in the coloring.

Once the cakes are cold, spread icing on top. Use candies and black writing icing to decorate them to look like animals. If you are planning ahead for a party, the cakes can be made up to a month in advance and frozen (uniced) in a plastic container. Thaw at room temperature before icing and decorating.

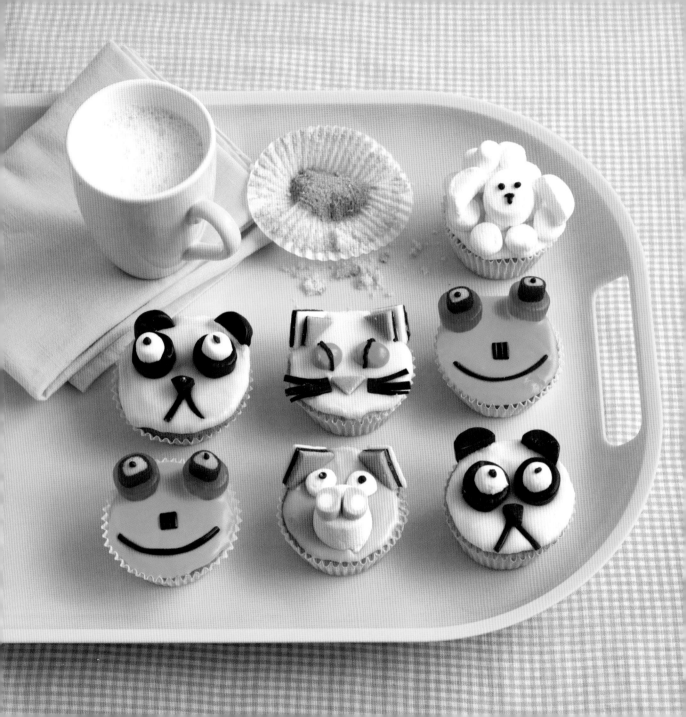

Annabel's Rice Krispies Squares ☺ ☹

What child, or adult for that matter, doesn't love Rice Krispies Squares? And they take only a few minutes to prepare. This is also a fun and easy recipe for children to make themselves. Keep the squares stored in the refrigerator until you are ready to eat them. You can use any combination of dried fruit, and dried mango is also good.

MAKES 9 SQUARES

4 oz white chocolate
5 tablespoons butter
3 tablespoons golden syrup (such as Lyle's) or light corn syrup
3 cups Rice Krispies
½ cup chopped mixed, dried fruits of your choice – try 3 tablespoons each
  chopped dried apricots, raisins, and dried cranberries

Break the chocolate into pieces and put into a saucepan, together with the butter and syrup, and melt over a low heat. Put the Rice Krispies and dried fruit into a large bowl and stir in the melted white-chocolate mixture.

Line a fairly shallow 8-inch square cake pan. Spoon the mixture into the pan and level the surface by pressing down gently with a potato masher. Place in the refrigerator to set and cut into squares before serving. Store in the refrigerator.

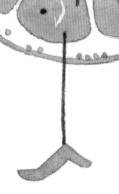

Yogurt and Raisin Cupcakes ❄ ☺ ☹

The yogurt and ground almonds keep these cupcakes lovely and moist. If you like, you could spread the tops of the cakes with glacé icing, as in the Animal Cupcakes (page 198), although I prefer to leave them plain.

MAKES 12 CAKES

$^2/_3$ cup unflavored yogurt

3 eggs, lightly beaten

1 teaspoon vanilla extract

$^3/_4$ cup plus 1 tablespoon superfine sugar

1 cup plus 2 tablespoons self-rising flour, plus extra for dusting

1 cup plus 2 tablespoons almond flour

1 teaspoon baking powder

a good pinch of salt

11 tablespoons (1 stick plus 3 tablespoons) butter, melted

$^1/_2$ cup raisins

Preheat the oven to 375°F. Line a 12-cup muffin pan with paper liners.

Put the yogurt, eggs, and vanilla extract in a small bowl and mix together. In a large bowl, whisk together the sugar, flour, almond flour, baking powder, and salt and make a well in the center. Pour in the yogurt mixture and the melted butter and quickly fold in the dry ingredients. Take care not to overmix. Finally, dust the raisins with a little flour and fold into the mixture.

Spoon the batter into the muffin cups. They will be quite full. Bake for 18–20 minutes or until risen and springy to the touch. Cool for a few minutes and then transfer to a wire rack to cool completely.

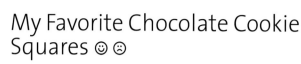

My Favorite Chocolate Cookie Squares ☺ ☹

These are great for a children's party or teatime treat. You could use just milk chocolate or plain chocolate if you prefer, and you could use only graham crackers. You can also substitute some mini marshmallows for the dried apricots.

MAKES 16 CHOCOLATE COOKIE SQUARES
8 sheets graham crackers
14 thin ginger snaps
3/4 cup milk chocolate chips
1/2 cup bittersweet chocolate chips
1/4 cup golden syrup, such as Lyle's
3/4 stick unsalted butter
1 cup ready-to-eat dried apricots, chopped
1/2 cup raisins
1 1/3 cups Rice Krispies

Lightly grease and line an 8-inch square shallow pan. Break the graham crackers and ginger snaps into large pieces, place in a plastic bag, and crush with a rolling pin to form coarse crumbs.

Melt the chocolate, syrup, and butter in a heatproof bowl over a saucepan of simmering water. Alternatively, melt in a microwave on High for 2 1/2–3 minutes, stirring halfway through. Stir in the cookie crumbs until well coated, then add the chopped apricots and raisins and, finally, stir in the Rice Krispies.

Spoon the mixture into the prepared pan. Level the surface, pressing down with a masher, and put in the refrigerator to set. Cut into squares before serving.

Index

About the author

Annabel Karmel is a mother of three and author of 22 bestselling books on feeding babies and children (as well as teaching children how to cook). Her books have sold over 4 million copies worldwide. She is well known for providing advice and guidance for millions of parents all over the world on what to feed their children, as well as getting families to eat a healthier diet without spending hours in the kitchen. Annabel travels frequently to the United States and has appeared on many TV shows including *The View*, *Live with Regis and Kelly*, and the *Today* show.

In 2006, Annabel was awarded an MBE (Member of the British Empire) by Queen Elizabeth for her services to nutrition for children and, in 2010, she won the media category of the First Women Awards, which recognize women at the top of their professions who are leading the way for the next generation. Her website, www.annabelkarmel.com, has more than 100,000 members and offers parents delicious recipes for babies, children, and adults, as well as information on all aspects of nutrition. She also has a successful iPhone app, "Annabel Karmel's Essential Guide to Feeding your Baby & Toddler" and a popular kids' cooking TV show, *Annabel's Kitchen*, which is loved by moms and kids, as well as a range of healthy Disney snacks for toddlers.

Acknowledgments

I am indebted to the following people for their help and advice during the writing of this book:

Margaret Lawson, Senior Lecturer in Pediatric Nutrition, Institute of Child Health, London; Professor Charles Brook, Consultant Pediatric Endocrinologist, Middlesex Hospital, UK; Dr. Sam Tucker FRCP, Consultant Pediatrician, Hillingdon Hospital, UK; Dr. Adam Fox MA (Hons), MSc, MB, BS, DCH, FRCPCH, FHEA, Pediatric Allergy Consultant, Evelina Children's Hospital.

Thanks also to: Jacqui Morley; Mary Jones; Caroline Stearns; and all the babies and their parents who helped with the photography for this edition. Everyone at Ebury Press, especially Sarah Lavelle, Vicky Orchard, Carey Smith, and Fiona Macintyre; Smith & Gilmour for their lovely design; Dave King for his beautiful photography; Nadine Wickenden for the gorgeous illustrations. My mother, Evelyn Etkind, for all her encouragement in writing this book. David Karmel, for his patience in teaching me how to use a computer. And, most important of all, my children, Nicholas, Lara, and Scarlett, for inspiring me to write this book.

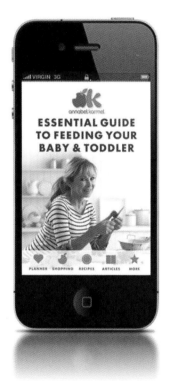